Breast Cancer

Breast Cancer

Web Resource Guide for Consumers, Healthcare Providers, Patients, and Physicians

Eugene A. De Felice, M.D.

Writers Club Press
San Jose   New York   Lincoln   Shanghai

Breast Cancer
Web Resource Guide for Consumers,
Healthcare Providers, Patients, and Physicians

Writers Club Press
an imprint of iUniverse, Inc.

For information address:
iUniverse, Inc.
5220 S. 16th St., Suite 200
Lincoln, NE 68512
www.iuniverse.com

ISBN: 0-595-22651-5

DEDICATION

This book is dedicated to Ms. Maryanne Harvey, M.S., Section Chief, Bureau of Environmental Radiation Protection, responsible for the mammography and radiation protection programs established and administered by the New York State Department of Health. Ms. Harvey is widely recognized for her many contributions to the field of mammography and radiology and also serves as Chairperson for the National Mammography Quality Assurance Advisory Committee of the U.S. Food and Drug Administration. Without Ms. Harvey's friendship, encouragement, dedication, contributions and able assistance in preparing and editing the manuscript, publication of this book would not have been possible.

CONTENTS

PREFACE

Most people do not pay sufficient attention to their health. Rather they tend to:

> Squander health in search of wealth
> They work and toil and save
> Then squander wealth in search of health
> But find an early grave.
>
> Anonymous

To prevent breast cancer, or to overcome it once it has occurred, one needs to become concerned, knowledgeable, and:

> Take charge, control, and responsibility for their health,
> Obtain reliable information about breast cancer,
> Follow steps to prevent occurrence whenever possible,
> Seek early detection if it can't be prevented, and
> Obtain effective treatment as soon as possible.

First, one needs to ask the right questions and obtain current, comprehensive and useful (CCU) information in order to become knowledgeable. In this regard, it has been said:

> I keep six honest serving men
> They taught me all I know
> Their names are What and Why and When

And How and Where and Who.
> Rudyard Kipling

Next, an intelligent person should want to know all there is to know about breast cancer and profit accordingly. To do otherwise is just not in one's best interests. A great leader in the field of breast cancer once said:

> I have always believed that intelligent people—not only wish
> to know as much as possible about any ailment they may have,
> but also that such people are entitled to know everything
> that is known about such ailments.
>> George Crile, M.D.

The Internet/Web provides the way to obtain easily accessible CCU breast cancer information. Many Web resources are available from which to obtain almost all, if not all, the information and expert opinion that one may need to become knowledgeable. In fact, it is now widely recognized that:

> Healthcare is not what it used to be
> Healthcare is not even what it ought to be
> Healthcare on the Web has grown to be
> Healthcare available for all as it should be
>> Eugene A. De Felice, M.D.

This book provides a very helpful guide to quickly and easily search the Web to obtain CCU breast cancer information. With such, one can take charge, control and responsibility for their health and can make informed decisions with their physician/healthcare provider and live a healthier, longer, happier and more enjoyable life.

Chapters I-7 address various aspects of female breast cancer. Chapter I is devoted to an introduction to breast cancer, statistics and anatomy. Chapter 2 covers risk factors and prevention. Chapter 3 discusses screening methods and diagnosis. Chapter 4 outlines stages and types of breast cancer. Chapter 5 explains treatments available. Chapter 6 is on ways to cope. Chapter 7 provides information on clinical trials. Chapter 8 concerns male breast cancer. Chapter 9 suggests useful ways of searching the Web. Chapter 10 presents the Author's List of Useful Web Resources and the information contained in each.

There is no one best answer for questions/issues concerning breast cancer. One must ultimately obtain the best information available and decide what is right under their particular circumstances of the moment in conjunction/consultation with their physician/healthcare provider.

It is estimated that well over 100 million Americans now consult the Web for healthcare information and the vast majority find it useful. I trust you will, too.

Eugene A. De Felice, M.D.

ACKNOWLEDGEMENTS

The author wishes to acknowledge that the Web Resources listed in Chapter 10, particularly the National Cancer Institute, were used as sources for the breast cancer information contained in this book. *Susan Love's Breast Book* by Susan M. Love, M.D.; *The Breast Cancer Wars: Hope, Fear and the Pursuit of a Cure in Twentieth Century American*, by Barron Lerner, M.D., *and Mammography and Beyond*, by Nass, Hendlers and Lashoff, also provided useful information and are highly recommended for further readings.

Special appreciation is afforded to my brother and literary agent, Benjamin De Felice, a "man for all seasons" and "helping hand to many" who was instrumental in arranging for the publication of this book.

CHAPTER 1

Introduction

1.1   Breast cancer

Breast cancer is a group of diseases that begin in the cells of the various breast structures, principally in the lobules and ducts. Breast structures are made up of different types of cells that normally grow and divide in an orderly, healthy manner and produce more cells only when the body needs them. However, sometimes, for reasons that remain to be clarified, breast cells keep dividing and growing abnormally in an uncontrolled fashion regardless of the body's needs, to form an independent mass of tissue called a growth or tumor. Such tumors can either be benign or malignant. Benign tumors are not cancer or life-threatening. They are localized, contain normal appearing cells, and usually can be removed easily and do not recur. Benign tumors do not spread or establish themselves in other parts of the body.

Malignant tumors are cancer and life threatening. These cancerous tumors contain cells that are abnormal in appearance and divide and grow in an uncontrolled, abnormal manner. Such abnormal cells can invade and damage nearby tissues. Also, such cancer cells can break away from the primary site in the breast, enter the blood stream or lymphatic system, and form new malignant tumors in other parts of the body. When breast cancer spreads outside the breast, cancer cells usually can be found in the lymph nodes under the arm and other organs. Spread of cancer cells in this way is called metastasis.

1.2   Statistics

Statistics help define the magnitude of the problem and relationship to other leading causes of death in the United States.

Breast cancer (BC) is reported to be the most common cancer among women excluding skin cancer. Around 192,200 new cases of invasive breast cancer were reported to have occurred in women in the United States in 2001. In comparison, only around 1,500 cases of breast cancer in men were diagnosed that year. Ductal carcinoma in situ (DCIS) accounted for around 40,000 new cases. DCIS is considered to be an early non-invasive form of breast cancer. Over 40,000 deaths from breast cancer occurred in women and 400 or so in men in the United States in 2001.

BC is the second leading cause of cancer death in women, exceeded only by lung cancer. Death rates from breast cancer are reported to have declined significantly in recent years, with the largest decreases occurring in younger women—both white and black. These decreases are believed to have occurred as a result of earlier detection and improved treatment.

About 1 in 8 women (12.5%) in the United States are expected to develop breast cancer during her lifetime. The National Cancer Institute estimates that a woman's chance of being diagnosed with breast cancer in any age group is approximately as follows:

Age Group	Chance of Being Diagnosed with Breast Cancer
30-40	1 in 257
40-50	1 in 67
50-60	1 in 36

60-70	1 in 28
70-80	1 in 24
in a lifetime	1 in 8

The following lifetime comparative risks for developing other common diseases places breast cancer in perspective:

Disease	Chance of Developing in a Lifetime
Heart Disease	1 in 2
Diabetes	1 in 3
Alcoholism	1 in 3
Stroke	1 in 5
Breast Cancer	1 in 8

Among the racial/ethnic groups evaluated, white, Hawaiian, and black women have the highest levels of breast cancer risk. Asian/Pacific Islander, and Hispanic women have a lower level of risk–their chance of developing breast cancer is less than two thirds of the risk of white women. The lowest level of breast cancer risk occurs among Korean, Native American, and Vietnamese women. These risks are population averages–an individual woman's risk may be higher or lower, depending upon a variety of factors, including family, reproductive history, and others.

1.3   Breast Anatomy

A basic knowledge of breast anatomy allows one to better understand breast cancer and its spread.

The human female breast consists of approximately 15 to 20 sections called lobes. Within each lobe are many smaller structures called lobules (milk producing glands) that end in dozens of very small bulbs that can produce milk. Lobes, lobules, and bulbs are all linked by thin tubes called ducts. These ducts lead to the nipple in the center of a darker colored area of the breast skin called areola. Stroma or connective tissue binds and supports breast structures and tissues. This connective tissue includes adipose (fat) tissue that gives the breast its softness, fibrous tissue for support, and blood and lymphatic vessels that carry the fluid that leaks out of the capillaries back into the blood circulatory system. This complex, colorless fluid that leaks out of the capillaries is collectively called lymph.

A series of lymph nodes (glandular structures) exist along the path of the lymph vessels and these constitute an integral part of the body's immune system involved in fighting and eliminating cancerous cells.

Lymph fluid from various structures in the breast is collected in the lymph plexus of Sappey in the nipple/ areola area and transported:

- Laterally via the lateral collecting truck to the subscapular and axilla (armpit) areas
- Medially via the medial collecting trunk to the intermammary nodes and the transmammary lymph pathway to the opposite breast
- Downward via the subdiaphragmatic pathway to the liver and intraabdominal nodes

The major lymphatic drainage of the breast is toward the axilla.

The lymph and blood circulatory systems are the pathways for spread or metastases of cancer cells to other organs/parts of the body.

Blockage or interruption of this complex lymphatic system of vessels and nodes/glands by surgery, radiation, or tumor cells leads to one of the major complications of breast cancer treatment, namely lymphedema, or an accumulation of lymph fluid and swelling in the axilla, arm and hand.

CHAPTER 2

Risk Factors and Prevention

Certain factors tend to expose a woman to a greater risk of developing breast cancer in her lifetime. These are called risk factors. They need to be taken into consideration in prevention, diagnosis and treatment.

Although risk factors are known to exist, and a woman has one or more, she will not necessarily develop breast cancer. Even if a woman has all the known risk factors, she still may never develop breast cancer in her lifetime. However, when one or more risk factors are present, the chances of developing breast cancer are increased.

While the majority of women have no known risk factors, the following are believed to increase the risk of a woman developing breast cancer:

- age–older women have a greater chance of occurrence. More than 3 out of 4 cases, and about 85 percent of deaths, occur in women over the age of 50
- birth control pills–use before age 20 or for more than 6 years
- breast disease–carcinoma in situ (CIS) or atypical hyperplasia (AH)
- bone density increase
- cancer history–past history of uterine, ovarian or colon cancer or a family history of breast cancer, especially in a mother or sister

- childbearing/pregnancy–never having had children or having children after age 30
- dense breast tissue–women older than 45 with at least 75 percent dense tissue on a mammogram
- failure to screen–failure to use early detection techniques and actions
- environmental exposure to smoke, pollutants, or chemicals, particularly those with estrogenic activity
- genetics–presence of BRCA-1, BRAC-2 or other cancer genes. Women with a family history of breast cancer who also have BRCA-1 have up to 50-85% lifetime risk.
- Hormone replacement therapy - with estrogen for 5 or more years
- Lifestyle factors
  - Alcohol - having more than 2 drinks daily
  - Chemical exposure - at home or work, especially to compounds that have estrogen like activity, e.g., pesticides
  - High fat diet
  - Obesity
  - Sedentary lifestyle
  - Smoking
- Menstruation beginning before age 12
- Menopause after age 55
- Pregnancy weight gain of 38 pounds or greater
- Race–white women have a slightly higher risk, black women a higher mortality, and Hispanic and Asian women have lower risk
- Radiation–substantial x-ray exposure, particularly to the chest wall during childhood and adolescence
- Shift work–working nights

- Surgery - involving breast reduction

Among these factors, the strongest appear to be:
- Family history—mother or sister diagnosed with the disease
- Previous breast biopsy showing atypical hyperplasia or carcinoma in situ

Patients taking certain preventative measures against key risk factors may decrease the risk of developing breast cancer. These preventative measures may include:
- Alcohol—decrease consumption to less than 2 drinks daily or discontinue drinking
- Birth control pills—use alternative methods or do not take them for more than 6 years
- Chemicals—avoid exposure in the environment or at work, especially to those with estrogen-like activity
- Childbearing—have children before age 30
- Failure to screen—employ routine breast exams and screening mammography
- High fat diet—reduce fat consumption to more normal levels
- Hormone replacement therapy—use alternative methods or limit to 5 years maximum
- Pregnancy weight gain—restrict to 30-35 pounds or less
- Radiation—reduce x-ray exposure to chest wall, particularly in younger females
- Sedentary lifestyle—adopt an active lifestyle and exercise regularly
- Smoking—stop entirely, avoid secondary smoke and environmental fumes

CHAPTER 3

Diagnosis

Generally, it is agreed that the earlier breast cancer is diagnosed, the better the chances of successful treatment outcome and survival.

Diagnosis is usually made initially on the basis of an evaluation of the following:

- History, symptoms and signs
- Breast self examination
- Clinical breast examination
- Mammography
- Film Screen Mammography (FSM)
- Full Field Digital Mammography (FFDM)
- Computer Aided Detection (CAD)
- Ultrasound Imaging (US)
- Magnetic Resonance Imaging (MRI

Most breast cancers are detected by FSM. Principally because of its lower cost as well as other considerations, FSM appears to be the only technology suitable at this time for general population breast screening examination (for early stages of beast cancer when the patient has no symptoms or signs of the disease). FFDM appears to be a major technical improvement over traditional FSM, however, it is not known at this time whether FFDM will lead to any better survival rate among screened women. CAD offers a means of improving accuracy of FSM in detection and is expected to become commonly used in the near future.

3.1   History, Symptoms and Signs

Certain patient/family history factors plus patient symptoms and signs are associated with development of breast cancer. When present, these should alert the patient and physician to the increased possibility of breast cancer being present, namely:

- Accentuated veins on breast surface
- Breast biopsy showing carcinoma in situ or atypical hyperplasia
- Breast size or shape change
- Crusting or scaling of the nipple
- Dimpling of breast skin resembling texture of an orange peel
- Discharge from nipple (clear to yellow or green, or bloody)
- Family history of breast cancer
- Lump or thickening in the breast/and or under the arm (axilla)
- Nipple inversion, retraction, enlargement, or persistent itching
- Redness or increased warmness of breast
- Sore or ulcer on skin of breast that does not heal readily
- Swelling of breast

A lump or thickening in the breast is usually the first sign of a possible breast tumor. Other symptoms and signs usually occur later in the development of breast cancer. Symptoms and signs of advanced disease may include bone pain, weight loss, swelling of one arm, and breast skin ulceration.

3.2   Breast Self-Examination

When a woman examines her own breasts for lumps and other changes, this is called breast self-examination (BSE).

Studies thus far have not shown that BSE alone reduces the death rate from breast cancer. Therefore, BSE should not be used alone or in place of clinical breast examination by a physician/healthcare provider.

Nevertheless, BSE is still considered to be useful for early detection of breast cancer, particularly in women properly instructed on how to do so, and especially in those women who do not receive an annual breast check up by their doctor.

It should be noted that around 80% of breast lumps not found on mammography are discovered by a woman who examines her own breasts. Also, when breast cancer is discovered early by a patient, when the lump is not too large, there may be a better survival and/or cosmetic result following surgical lumpectomy.

Information on the pros and cons of BSE, and recommended ways to conduct such examinations, may be found via the following four Web Resources:

- Cancer Research Foundation of American (CRFA)–http://www.crfa.org
- CNN.com (Cleveland Clinic)–http://www.cnn.com/health
- Komen Breast Center Foundation (KBCF)–http://www.komen.org
- Mayo Clinic–http://www.mayo.org

CRFA shows how to conduct a BSE in front of a mirror, lying down, and in the shower, and when to schedule the self-exam.

The Cleveland Clinic (CNN.com/Health) provides a concise and helpful BSE which can be used with a mirror, in the shower, or lying down, plus information on "What should I do if I find a lump?" Information site also is provided for "What to expect from your doctor's exam". The Cleveland Clinic also recommends a BSE monthly in women starting at age 20. For further information go to CNN.com, click on Health, then click on Breast Self Exam.

The KBCF has a Breast Self Exam Card in English or Spanish which illustrates the proper steps to be taken in a BSE.

The Mayo Patient Education Center also provides information on the pros and cons of the exam, and how to properly conduct, a BSE. At the Mayo Clinic, every woman is regarded as being at some risk of developing breast cancer in her lifetime. Therefore a BSE is recommended once a month beginning at age 20 and continuing throughout life supplemented with a clinical breast examination by a health professional every 3 years until age 40 and annually thereafter.

3.3   Clinical Breast Examination

A clinical breast examination (CBE) is performed by a physician/ healthcare provider once a year usually during an annual physical examination. During this examination, the physician/healthcare provider checks for lumps or other unusual changes in both breasts and under the arms (armpits). It is important that such CBEs be thorough and be done only by persons trained and experienced in such examinations.

The Cleveland Clinic Hospital recommends a CBE be done every 3 years starting at age 20 to 39, and every year from age 40 thereafter. CBEs may be done more often on women at high risk for breast cancer.

However, it should be recognized that there is insufficient clinical evidence available at this time to conclusively show that BSE or CBE alone significantly reduces the breast cancer death rate.

3.4   Mammography

A mammogram is a special low dose x-ray of the breast that often can find breast cancer tumors too small for the patient or the doctor to feel. Also, mammograms are useful for detecting calcium deposits that cannot be felt through palpation. While most such calcium deposits are of little clinical significance, a cluster of tiny specs of calcium, called microcalcifications may be associated with the presence of a small breast cancer and can alert the doctor accordingly.

The ability of a mammogram to detect early breast cancer depends on such factors as the size of the tumor, age of the patient, breast density, and the experience and skill of the radiologist. Studies have shown that screening mammography tends to be most useful in women over 50.

- Film Screen Mammography

FSM, otherwise known as traditional or conventional mammography, has been in use for many years now. It provides reasonably high quality images in the vast majority of patients at low radiation doses. However, FSM may not provide adequate diagnostic information for some patients, particularly those with dense breast tissue. In fact, it has been estimated that FSM misses about 15% of all breast cancers. It is often difficult for the radiologist to determine whether a suspicious finding on the mammogram is cancer or not.

From 60-85% of all lesions detected by FSM alone are benign (non-cancerous) and may lead to many unnecessary biopsies. Thus, technologies in addition to FSM are still needed to improve detection and diagnosis and a number are currently being investigated.

- Computer-Aided Detection

CAD is one such newer technology designed to complement FSM. The FDA recently approved CAD for diagnostic use in evaluating suspicious areas of the breast found using conventional FSM.

CAD systems scan mammograms with a laser beam and convert the result-ant image into a digital signal that is processed by a computer to identify possible cancerous lesions. Video monitors display the mammographic image with CAD markers highlighting suspicious areas. Thus, CAD serves as a "virtual second opinion" to the radiologist in reading a mammogram. Retrospective studies have shown that CAD decreases the rate of false-neg-ative readings (stating that a tumor is not present when it is).

It is estimated that over 30 million screening and 3 million diagnostic mammograms (FSMs) were performed in the United States in 2001. However, for every 80 breast cancers detected through routine screening mammograms in healthy women, an additional 20 cancers are not detected because they are overlooked or look benign. Thus, estimates indi-cate that for every 100,000 breast cancers currently detected by FSMs, adding CAD use (in addition) could result in the early detection of an additional 20,000 plus breast cancers (20% more). Such CAD improved detection of early stage disease would be expected to result in better sur-vival and decreased mortality from breast cancer over time.

- Full Field Digital Mammography

FFDM uses a detector that responds to x-rays passing through breast tissue by sending an electronic signal to a computer to be digitalized and processed. The physician can change the film image contrast and magnification to improve his/her ability to identify lesions. FFDM is reported to facilitate CAD, tomosynthesis, and telemammography. Widespread use of FFDM currently is limited by cost and somewhat lower resolution as compared with FSM and CAD. The utility and place of FFDM in the screening and diagnosis of breast cancer remains to be established. A Digital Mammographic Imaging Screening Trial (DMIST) involving 50,000 or so patients in the United States and Canada sponsored by the American College of Radiology Imaging Network (ACRIN) and the National Cancer Institute (NCI) is currently underway to try to answer this question. The key objective of this study is to determine how well FFDM compares to FSM in terms of screening detection of breast cancer.

• Mammography Screening

A woman should consider having her first screening mammogram when she is about 10 years younger than the earliest age at which a first-degree relative has been diagnosed with breast cancer, or at age 40, whichever comes sooner. Women younger than 40 or over 69, and those at high risk, should seek medical advice regarding mammography screening.

The National Cancer Institute now recommends that a woman have a screening mammogram every 1-2 years starting at age 40.

It should be remembered that FSM may detect breast cancer some 2-5 years before it becomes large enough to be found clinically as a lump. Also, early detection may result in a significant reduction in death from breast cancer, particularly in women over age 50 and those at high risk.

Mammography is a screening tool with limitations. In women under 50 years of age, mammography is likely to miss 20-30% of existing breast cancers, and in women over 50, around 10%. Thus, when a woman and/or her doctor feel a suspicious breast lump that is not confirmed by mammography, the breast should be examined by some other means such as ultrsonography or magnetic resonance imaging. Also, mammography sometimes indicates a suspicious area in the breast when none exists. However, while false positives can be clarified by other procedures, this requires a repeat exam, possibly a biopsy, temporary anxiety, and additional costs. Also, mammograms do not appear to work as well in women taking hormone replacement therapy (HRT) which cause breasts to become more dense making mammograms more difficult to read.

Nevertheless, screening mammography remains the key to detecting breast cancer early–when it is small, less than one half inch in size. When detected/ diagnosed early and small, most patients will need only surgery and radiation without chemotherapy, and will have much less chance of dying from the disease. In contrast, if the breast cancer is detected when it is as big as a quarter (2.5 centimeters or an inch or so in size), patients usually have to undergo more extensive surgery, radiation, and chemotherapy, etc. and the death rate may rise accordingly to 20-25% and more. Thus, the maxim for breast cancer is "find it early and small".

3.5   Magnetic Resonance Imaging

MRI is a method of imaging tissue where atoms in a strong magnetic field absorb pulses of radiowaves and emit characteristic signals that are analyzed by computer. These signals vary according to the tissue type (e.g., fat, muscle, fibrous and edema fluid.) MRI is reported to cause minimal hazards from magnetic field effects and to be reasonably safe. It does not use any ionizing radiation and is free of any such health effects.

MRI, like FSM, is used to find structural abnormalities in breast tissue. Breast tumors show increased tissue uptake of the contrast agent used and are differentiated accordingly.

MRI was developed primarily as a diagnostic tool to reduce the incidence of unnecessary breast biopsies, especially in women having dense breast tissue and lesions difficult to detect properly using FSM.

While MRI has generally been considered to be too expensive for routine population screening, applications of a screening nature are still being evaluated, particularly among high risk populations.

Potential advantages of MRI over FSM include better detection of: 1) multiple malignancies, 2) invasive lobular carcinoma, 3) recurrent cancers, and 4) breast cancers in high risk patients having dense breast tissue.

Liabilities of MRI include: 1) a lack of uniform interpretation criteria regarding images/results, 2) low ability to detect microcalcifications and very small tumors especially if they do not pick up the contrast agent used, and 3) expense.

3.6   Ultrasonography

US uses high frequency sound waves that reflect boundaries between tissues with different acoustic properties in order to create an image called a sonogram. It is used principally to evaluate breast lumps that have been identified by mammography in order to differentiate a benign cyst from a solid tumor since a fluid-filled cyst gives rise to a different "sound signature". US is regarded as having poor ability to detect microcalcifications associated with small breast cancers due to a phenomena called "speckle". Combining imaging techniques may help reduce interference from "speckling" and is the subject of ongoing research in the field. However, at this time, studies have shown that US alone is not a useful screening tool for breast cancer.

However, US is a well established adjunct to mammography as a method to:

- Diagnose breast cysts
- Localize tumors
- Guide aspiration and biopsy needles

Several more recent studies suggest that US may be more widely used in the future to:

- Characterize tumors as benign versus malignant
- Screen for more specific high risk populations

3.7   *Mammography and Beyond*

Mammography and Beyond: Developing Technologies for the Early Detection of Breast Cancer, published by the Institute of Medicine and the National Research Council in 2001 provides a status report with detailed information on mammography and other technologies available and under development for the early detection of breast cancer. Interested readers may review this book online in its entirety through the National Academy Press website at: http://www.nap.edu.

3.8   Breast Biopsy/Aspiration

Should a clinical breast exam and/or mammogram reveal a suspicious lesion, patients usually are advised to have an aspiration and/or biopsy to determine if the lesion is cancer. Depending on circumstances, the following procedures, among others, may be employed to arrive at a diagnosis:

- Fine needle biopsy/aspiration

This procedure is performed with a fine needle under local anesthesia to remove fluid and/or cells from a breast tumor to be checked by a pathologist for cancer cells. If the fluid obtained is clear, it may not need to be checked further. If no cancer cells or infection are found, then a diagnosis of a benign breast cyst can be made.

• Core needle biopsy

This involves removing breast tissue with a larger needle under local anesthesia from an area that looks suspicious on a mammogram or an ultrasound, and can or cannot be felt. The tissue is evaluated by a pathologist for the presence of abnormal cells, e.g., atypical hyperplasia or cancerous cells.

• Surgical biopsy

Under local or general anesthesia, a surgeon cuts out a sample of a lump or suspicious area of the affected breast. In an excisional biopsy, the surgeon removes the entire lump or suspicious area plus some healthy surrounding tissues. In both cases, a pathologist then examines the removed tissue under a microscope to check for atypical hyperplasia or cancerous cells in order to establish a diagnosis.

3.9   Biomarkers

Biomarkers are characteristics of cancer cells that can be measured with sophisticated biological tests. They are used to help differentiate cancer types and evaluate how aggressively they may behave, as well as their response to treatment. A number of these biomarkers are now currently in use. These include, among others: 1) estrogen and progesterone receptor tests, 2) Her-2 neu oncogene receptor test, 3) S-phase fraction test and 4) ploidy test.

• Estrogen and Progesterone Receptor Tests

This is one of the most common and useful of the biomarkers tests. Cancers that are sensitive to estrogen and/or progesterone–that have these receptors–usually are somewhat slower growing and have slightly better prognosis than tumors without them. Cancers that are estrogen receptor negative but progesterone receptor positive usually still respond to hormone blocking drugs such as tamoxifen and the aromatase inhibitor class of drugs (discussed in Chapter 5.6). Also, this test indicates whether a given cancer can be successfully treated with a hormonal blocking agent such as tamoxifen or an aromatase inhibitor. Cancers sensitive to estrogen and/or progesterone usually show a positive response, and those that are not, rarely respond to such hormone blocking drugs. Postmenopausal women with breast cancer tend to be more likely to have estrogen receptor positive and premenopausal women are more likely to be estrogen receptor negative.

• Her-2 Neu Oncogene Receptor Test

Her-2 is an example of a dominant oncogene that is overexpressed in about one third of invasive breast cancers. Having a breast cancer tested for Her-2 receptor is considered to be useful for determining:

- Aggressiveness or propensity of the cancer to invade, spread, and metastasize
- Most useful treatment. Her-2 positive cancers appear to respond well to adriamycin, for example.
- Whether a patient with metastatic breast cancer is a candidate for Herceptin, a monoclonal blocking antibody to the Her-2 receptor
- Whether Herceptin may be useful as adjuvant therapy in earlier stages I-III invasive breast cancer

- S-phase Fraction Test

This test is used to determine how rapidly breast cancer cells are dividing and growing. The S-phase fraction is the percentage of cells that are dividing at any one time assessed by computer analysis. A high S-phase fraction indicates that the tumor may be behaving more aggressively. A low S-phase fraction is taken to indicate less aggressiveness and a better prognosis and survival. The main use of the S-phase fraction test lies in deciding which node negative breast cancers may need further treatment and which may not.

- Ploidy Test

Ploidy refers to the amount of DNA that cancer cells have within them. When cells have the normal amount of DNA, they are called diploid, and when the amount is abnormal, they are called aneuploid. Aneuploid tumors are reported to account for around 70% of breast cancers. Diploid tumors are regarded as less aggressive whereas aneuploid cancers are considered to be more aggressive.

3.10   Genetic Testing

The value of genetic breast cancer testing for the vast majority of women remains to be established.

Breast Cancer is more common in women with a family history of the disease suggesting certain genetic factors may be operative. Approximately 5-10% of all women with breast cancer are estimated to have a germ-line mutation of the genes, BRCA1 and BRCA2, associated with the development of breast cancer. Such mutations are reported to be more common in women of Jewish ancestry than in other ethnic groups.

BRCA1 gene, discovered in 1991, is a tumor suppressor gene linked to both genetic breast and ovarian cancers. Women/families who have this gene are reported to suffer from a high incidence of breast cancer, often at an early age, and in both breasts as well as from ovarian cancer.

BRCA2 gene, discovered in 1994, is less common and carries less cancer risk than BRCA1.

While BRCA1 affects only women, BRCA2 can also affect men. The risk of ovarian cancer carried by BRCA 2 also is lower than that of BRCA1.

These mutations also are associated with an increased risk of primary cancer elsewhere in the body.

In women who test positive for the BRCA1 and BRCA2 genetic breast cancer markers, the estimated lifetime risk of developing breast cancer appears to range from 50- 85%.

Genetic testing currently is available to detect BRCA1 and BRCA2 mutations in women who are considered to be at high risk for developing breast cancer. However, women considering such tests should weigh all the known benefits and limitations of such early knowledge and seek/be referred to counseling beforehand.

It should be noted that, among other considerations, genetic testing is expensive. Future insurance/employment discrimination may prove to be a problem for patients who test positive. The impact on other family members also needs to be taken into consideration. And the best way to treat patients with positive test results remains to be clarified.

For further information on genetic testing, the reader may look to the National Cancer Institute (http://www.cancer.gov) or one or more of the other appropriate Web Resources listed in Chapter 10.

CHAPTER 4

Stages/Types of Cancer

Once a diagnosis of breast cancer is established, staging/classification usually is determined to help guide future treatment and follow-up.

The International Union Against Cancer (IUAC) and the American Joint Committee on Cancer (AJCC) have developed a 5 stage standardized system of describing and staging newly diagnosed breast cancer cases known as TNM. The letter "T" involves the cancer's size, "N" indicates whether or not the surrounding lymph nodes contain cancer cells and "M" concerns whether or not the cancer has spread/metastasized to other organs/parts of the body such as lungs, bones, liver, brain, etc. All this information is combined in a prescribed fashion and then used to determine a patient's overall cancer stage in Roman numerals from 0 (earliest) to IV (advanced). While this TNM system has limitations, it is still considered useful. However, the key factor regarding breast cancer prognosis still remains whether or not the tumor has spread to other organs as this ultimately determines in a large measure who lives or dies.

The AJCC defines breast cancer stages as follows:
- Stage 0–in situ (in place) disease in which cancerous cells are in their location of origin within normal breast tissue

- Stage I–tumor less than 2 centimeters in diameter with no spread beyond the breast
- Stage IIA–tumor 2-5 centimeters in size without spread to axillary lymph nodes, or tumor less than 2 centimeters in size with spread to axillary lymph nodes
- Stage IIB–tumor greater than 5 centimeters in size without spread to axillary lymph nodes, or tumor 2-5 centimeters in size with spread to axillary lymph nodes
- Stage IIIA–tumor smaller than 5 centimeters with spread to axillary lymph nodes which are attached to each other or to other structures, or tumor greater than 5 centimeters with spread to axillary lymph nodes
- Stage IIIB–tumor has invaded the breast skin, chest wall, or has spread to lymph nodes inside the chest wall along the sternum
- Stage IV–a tumor of any size with spread beyond the region of the breast and chest wall, such as to the liver, bone, lungs or other organs. This is regarded as metastatic breast cancer.

Stage 0, carcinoma in situ, involves two main types:

- Lobular carcinoma in situ

  LCIS is regarded as a noninvasive lobular neoplasm beginning in a breast lobule (milk producing gland) and consists of abnormal cells existing only in the lining of the lobule. While such abnormal cells usually don't develop into invasive cancer, their presence is believed to indicate an increased risk of breast cancer in both breasts over the long term. Patients with this diagnosis may choose not to have further treatment or take medication that may help prevent development of breast cancer.

- Ductual carcinoma in situ

DCIS is a noninvasive ductal neoplasm with cancer cells in the lining of a duct of a lobule that have not spread to surrounding breast tissue. DCIS accounts for around 20-25% of all breast cancers. Almost all DCIS are reported to be detectable by mammograms and are uncommonly found by breast self-examination by the patient or clinical breast examination by a physician. While DCIS is usually noninvasive, it may spread over time. Therefore, patients with this diagnosis may elect to have breast-sparing surgery followed by radiation or more aggressive therapy.

Stages I and II are considered to be early stages of invasive/infiltrating breast cancer. Chief examples include:

• Invasive ductal carcinoma (IDC)

These breast cancers start in the milk ducts, spread through the duct wall, invade surrounding fatty tissue/stroma, and have the potential to spread to other parts of the body/organs via the lymphatic and/or blood circulatory systems. IDC is the most common form of breast cancer accounting for about 70-80% of all breast malignancies.

• Invasive lobular carcinoma (ILC)

Such breast cancers arise in the milk producing glands or lobules, invade surrounding breast fatty tissue and stroma, and have the potential to spread elsewhere in the body. ILC constitutes about 10-15% of all invasive breast cancers and is often difficult to detect by patient breast self-examination or physician clinical breast examination, or even mammography.

Stage III is regarded as a more advanced form of breast cancer than earlier stages I and II.

Stage IV is metastatic breast cancer and occurs when breast cancer has spread to other parts of the body.

Miscellaneous and less common forms of breast cancer, among others, include:

• Medullary carcinoma (MC)

  MC is a special type of invasive breast cancer with a well-defined border between normal and cancerous tissue accounting for up to 5% of all breast cancers. The long term survival for this type of breast cancer is considered to be better than for most other invasive breast cancers.

• Inflammatory Breast Cancer (IBC)

  IBC is a rare type of breast cancer accounting for only around 1% of all invasive tumors. IBC usually is quite aggressive, spreads more or less rapidly to other organs/parts of the body and is difficult to treat. Usually the skin over the affected breast feels warm to touch, appears red in color, and becomes thickened to an orange-peel texture (peau d'orange) due to cancer cells blocking lymph vessels/channels in the skin of the affected breast.

• Paget's Disease of the Nipple (PDN)

  PDN invasive breast cancer starts in the milk ducts, involves both skin and nipple, and can spread to the areola. It accounts for only around

1% or so of all breast cancers. Patients usually exhibit crusting, scaly, red, inflamed tissue in the nipple area along with oozing, burning, or bleeding as the disease advances. It may be associated with ILC or IDC.

Other even rarer forms of breast tumors also may occur such as cytosarcoma phyllodes (from connective tissue), angiosarcoma (from blood vessels), lipoma or liposarcoma (from fatty tissue), and primary lymphoma (from lymph system). These can be local and benign, or invasive and malignant. However, they will not be dealt with further as they are considered to be outside the scope of this book.

CHAPTER 5

Treatment

5.1   Overview

Breast cancer treatment involves local, or both local and systemic therapy. Local treatment usually consists of surgery, or both surgery and radiation to take care of the cancer in the breast and surrounding lymph nodes, when involved. Surgery may consist of only removal of the breast lump - or partial, total or radical mastectomy. Special procedures (sentinel node biopsy) also may be used to find the most likely lymph node(s) to which the cancer may or may not have spread in order to try to limit therapy. Radiation therapy may be directed at the tumor, the breast, chest wall, or other tissues known or suspected to have remaining cancer cells. Systemic therapy includes chemotherapy, hormonal therapy, biological therapy or some combination of the three. Systemic therapy is used to help eliminate cancer cells that may remain in the breast or lymph system after surgery and radiation, and may have spread to other parts of the body.

Most patients with stage 0 are treated with surgery alone or surgery plus radiation. Patients with stage I-IV usually are treated with a combination of surgery, radiation, chemotherapy, hormonal therapy and biological therapy. Treatment added to surgery and radiation is called adjuvant therapy and is given to eliminate any remaining cancer cells.

For stages I-III, the main considerations are to adequately treat the breast cancer and prevent a recurrence either at the place of origin (local) or elsewhere in the body (metastases). For stage IV, the goal is to improve symptoms and prolong survival as long as possible. Stage IV cannot be "cured" in most cases; 5-year survival occurs in less than 15-20 % of cases.

5.2   Surgery

Surgery is the most common basic treatment for breast cancer. Different types of surgery may be employed.

- Types of Surgical Therapy

  An operation to remove the cancer and some surrounding normal tissue is called breast-sparing or breast-conserving surgery. Lumpectomy (removal of tumor mass and some surrounding normal tissue) and segmental mastectomy (partial mastectomy) are types of breast-conserving surgery that may be used. Sometimes an excisional biopsy may serve as a lumpectomy. Often, some of the lymph nodes under the arm may be removed at the time of the lumpectomy.

  When the entire involved breast is removed, this is called a simple mastectomy. If the surgeon also removes the lymph nodes under the arm to determine whether cancer cells have entered the lymphatic system and spread, this is called an axillary lymph node dissection.

  A modified radical mastectomy involves removing the whole breast and most, if not all, the lymph nodes under the arm, and, often the lining over the chest muscles. The smaller of the two chest muscles also may be removed to assist in the removal of lymph nodes.

In a radical mastectomy, the entire breast is removed along with both chest muscles, all of the lymph nodes under the arm, and some additional surrounding fat and skin.

- Lymphedema

  Lymphedema is a swelling caused by an accumulation of lymph fluid in the axilla, arm and hand on the affected side which occurs in 10-15% or more cases following mastectomy, under arm lymph node dissection and/or radiation therapy. Under normal circumstances, lymph fluid moves into lymph vessels and nodes, and returns to the blood stream unimpeded. However, after removal of lymph nodes and vessels by surgery or destruction by radiation, passage of lymph fluid into the blood stream is interrupted and accumulates in the axilla, arm and hand on the affected side. In certain cases, it can be so slight that the patient notices it because fingers swell and the ring on the ring finger is tight fitting and not easily removed, or the swelling becomes so severe that the arm becomes huge. It can occur immediately or months or years after the operation, and it can be temporary, if lymph vessels and nodes regenerate, or permanent, if they do not.

  It usually proceeds through 4 stages. Stage 0 or the latency stage, refers to the period in which the arm is not swollen to any significant degree. Stage 1 occurs when there is a reversible, soft swelling and the skin over the swelling is still normal. Stage 2 is no longer spontaneously reversible because fibrous changes in the tissues have occurred to make the arm feel somewhat hard. Finally, in Stage 3, "lymphostatic elephantiasis" occurs where there is an extreme increase in volume of the affected arm, and skin changes, including deep skin folds appear.

  While there is no cure for lymphedema, there is some treatment that can improve the condition. Patients need to act early and aggressively to treat the condition even when there is only a small amount of fluid accumulation observed in order to achieve best results. Therapy may consist of: 1) elevation of the arm with pillows to reduce swelling, 2) elastic cuff to improve lymph circulation, 3) use of a support glove, 4) physical therapy, 5) manual massage, 6) exercise, 7) a pump to gently compress the arm. Some useful combination of procedures 1-7 may be employed to reverse the condition before it becomes irreversible and severe.

- Sentinel Node Biopsy

Removal of all visible lymph nodes under the arm does not appear to improve survival in breast cancer patients. However, it is usually done to: 1) determine if the cancer has spread, 2) prevent recurrence in the armpit, and 3) decide on adjuvant systemic chemotherapy. Unfortunately, radical lymph node removal in the armpit often results in complications such as lymphedema.

Sentinel node biopsy has been proposed as a better way to determine if the breast cancer has spread, avoiding the complications of more radical removal of lymph nodes. Sentinel nodes are a limited set of lymph nodes in the axilla to which breast cancer is most likely to spread first. In sentinel node biopsy, only one or a few lymph nodes are removed for laboratory analysis for cancer cells by a pathologist when a patient has a lumpectomy or mastectomy.

In this procedure, a small amount of a blue dye and/or radioactive material is injected into the breast at the site of the breast cancer. This injected material drains to the nearby lymphatic system to the first lymph node(s) for that area of the breast. It is presumed that this node(s) is also the most likely to have drained any cancer cells from the breast cancer. This first draining node(s), the sentinel node, is then surgically removed and examined by a pathologist for cancer cells. If the sentinel node is free of cancer cells, it is believed that there is a very low chance that there are any cancer cells in other lymph nodes.

The usefulness of this procedure remains controversial at this time. The impact of removing only the sentinel node(s) has on cancer control and survival remains to be established. It is not known if it can safely replace more radical surgery involving removal of all lymph nodes in the armpit area.

The National Cancer Institute is now sponsoring two clinical trials to try to answer these questions. One study is being conducted by the National Surgical Adjuvant Breast and Bowel Project (NSABP) to determine if sentinel node biopsy can replace axillary node dissection in patients with negative sentinel nodes. The other trial is being conducted by the American College of Surgeons in women with positive sentinel nodes to determine if it can replace removal of all axillary lymph nodes. These studies are currently in progress but years away from completion.

5.3   Breast Reconstruction

For patients having a mastectomy, reconstructive surgery may be employed at the time of surgery (immediate reconstruction) or at some subsequent time (delayed reconstruction). Breast contour/shape can be restored by the submuscular insertion of an artificial implant (saline-filled), a rectus muscle, or other muscle flap. In cases where a saline implant is used, a tissue expander can be inserted beneath the pectoral muscle. Saline is then injected into the expander to stretch tissues over a period of weeks or months until the desired size/shape, volume is obtained. The tissue expander subsequently is replaced by a more permanent implant.

While current evidence indicates that silicone implants do not cause breast cancer or autoimmune disease, they are available only through restricted clinical trials.

Rectus muscle flaps require a considerably more complicated and prolonged operative procedure and blood transfusions not uncommonly may be required.

Further information on implants may be obtained online from the U.S. Food and Drug Administration at: http://www.fda.gov.

5.4   Radiotherapy

Radiation therapy (RT) uses high energy x-rays to kill breast cancer cells locally in the breast as well as lymph nodes in the affected area. This ionizing radiation injures or destroys cells in the area being treated by damaging their genetic material making it impossible for the cells to continue to divide, grow, and function normally. While radiation damages both cancer and normal cells, the latter are able to undergo repair and recover and function normally again.

The type of radiation commonly used involves photons or packets of energy. X-rays were the first form of photon radiation used to treat cancer. The higher the energy of the x-ray beam, the deeper the x-rays can go into the target tissue.

Most hospitals and clinics now use external radiation generated by electricity. The machine used to do this is called a linear accelerator that produces the x-ray beam aimed directly at the cancerous tissue site. The beam of x-ray photons generated is sharpened in focus in the head of the machine to increase accuracy and minimize scatter and the potential to harm surrounding normal tissue.

Another less common way to administer RT is to place radioactive implants directly in a tumor site such as after a lumpectomy. This is called brachytherapy.

The RT treatment plan depends on a number of factors including the hospital or clinic facilities, the surgeon, oncologist, breast cancer type and spread and patient preferences, among others.

RT is principally used as localized treatment in conjunction with surgery to improve outcome/survival. The goal of surgery is to remove the cancer so that it will not recur in the breast, surgical scar or chest wall. This usually is done by removing as much as possible of breast cancer tissue via a lumpectomy, segmental (partial) mastectomy, or total mastectomy. The goal of RT is to destroy any remaining cancer cells in the region and surrounding lymph nodes/system. In principle, RT can be done either at the time of surgery or later as the case may indicate. Sometimes, when the tumor is large, RT may be done prior to surgery to shrink the tumor and facilitate removal.

Lumpectomy and RT together appear to produce about the same survival rate from breast cancer and almost the same local recurrence rate as mastectomy. Available results indicate that after 12 years, lumpectomy alone results in a local recurrence rate of around 35%, lumpectomy plus RT a 10% rate and mastectomy an 8% rate.

Women who choose lumpectomy instead of the more disfiguring mastectomy surgery for their breast cancer typically receive daily radiation beam therapy for 5 weeks to help prevent cancer recurrence. A recent study in 1200 Canadian women for 5 years indicates that cutting that schedule to

3 weeks appears to work equally well. Women who received the shortened radiation schedule had the same low rate of recurrence of around 3% as the long radiation schedule even though the total amount of radiation given was roughly equal in both groups.

Side effects, such as thickening of breast tissue, appearance of small blood vessels, and other effects, were found to be comparable in both groups, occurring in less than 25% of patients.

The new shorter duration schedule means 10 fewer trips to the hospital/clinic for patients and substantial savings for health care providers. Also, the shorter schedule lessens the burden for women with breast cancer in terms of convenience and personal costs in terms of travel, time off from work, and financial expenses.

5.5   Chemotherapy

Chemotherapy (CT) is adjuvant drug therapy used in addition to surgery and radiation to kill cancer cells that may remain or may have spread to the surrounding lymph nodes or other organs/parts of the body. The drugs used may be given in a pill form by mouth or by injection. Most patients have chemotherapy in an outpatient part of a hospital or clinic, at the doctor's office, or at home. Depending on drugs used and other factors, patients may need to stay in the hospital during at least a part of such treatment.

• Standard Chemotherapy Regimens

CT usually involves a combination of drugs which are regarded as useful for most pre- and post-menopausal patients regardless of lymph node involvement or estrogen and progesterone receptor status. Some of these regimens may include:

AC = doxorubicin (Adriamycin), cyclophosphamide

AT = doxorubicin (Adriamycin), docetaxel (Taxol)

ACT = AC followed by Taxol

CAF = cyclophosphamide, Adriamycin, 5-fluorouracil

CEF = cyclophosphamide, epirubicin, 5-fluorouracil

CMF = cyclophosphamide, methrotrexate, 5-fluorouracil

Cyclophosphamide, methotrexate, and 5-fluorouracil are well established chemotherapeutic agents for the treatment of breast cancer.

The anthracyclines, (doxorubicin and epirubicin) and the taxanes, (paclitaxel and docetacel) are newer additions to the standard CT regiments that have been found to be useful in the treatment of breast cancer. Further information on the indications, efficacy, safety and side effects of these CT drugs, as well as all others, may be obtained from the Food and Drug Administration at http://www.fda.gov.

Adriamycin appears to be one of the most effective drugs available, especially for metastatic breast cancer. However, it is associated with significant cardiotoxicity. Epirubicin, a newer, close chemical relative, may be considered preferable from a safety standpoint since it appears to have a lower cardiotoxicity potential. The taxanes, paclitaxel (Taxol) and docetaxel (Taxotere), also appear to show promise in the treatment of breast cancer.

At this time it is not known whether a single agent or combination of drugs is preferable for first line treatment of breast cancer. Also, combinations of CT and hormonal therapy have not shown a significant overall survival advantage over sequential use of these agents. And, the optimal combination of available drugs for CT, or hormonal therapy, of any given type of breast cancer or stage remains to be established.

Overall results in invasive breast cancer with existing CT indicate that:

- For patients under 50 years of age, combination CT is associated with 10-year survival of around 80% for those with node-negative disease, and approximately 50% with node-positive disease

- For patients 50-69 years of age, a 10-year survival of around 70% for those with node-negative disease and 45-50% with node positive disease.

Anthracycline-containing CT regimens appear to have a slight advantage in terms of survival in both pre- and post-menopausal patients. Also, there is some evidence to suggest that there may be particular tumor characteristics predicting anthracycline responsiveness.

CT often may involve serious short and long-term side effects and complications such as: hair loss, premature menopause, infertility, weight gain, memory loss, fatigue, bone marrow suppression and infection, cardiotoxicity, and even death, among others. Further information on side effects and complications is available from the NCI in a report online entitled: "What You Need to Know About Breast Cancer" (sections entitled "Side Effects of Treatment" and "Chemotherapy and You") at http://www.cancer.gov.

- Anthracyclines (doxorubicin, epirubicin)

There are two major anthracyclines available for the treatment of breast cancer that has spread to the lymph nodes. One is doxorubicin (Adriamycin) that has been available for a number of years and is considered to be one of the better chemotherapeutic agents available. The other is epirubicin (Ellence) which was approved in September 1999 also for the treatment of early stage invasive breast cancer that has spread to the lymph nodes under the arm and that has been treated surgically to remove all known tumor.

The anthracyclines interfere with a number of biological and biochemical functions within cancer cells leading to their destruction although the precise mechanism of action is not completely understood. Both of these anthracyclines are commonly used in combination with other chemotherapeutic agents to treat patients with breast cancer to slow or halt the progression of the disease and prolong life.

An epirubicin containing combination, CEF, recently was reported to have produced a significantly increased 5-year survival rate without relapse compared to the standard combination, CMF (62% vs. 53%), and increased 5-year overall survival (77% vs. 70%) compared to those given CMF therapy. At higher doses, CEF produced a significantly greater 5-year survival without relapse (65% vs. 52%), and a 5-year overall survival of 76% vs. 65% compared to those patients given the lower dose of epirubicin.

Results to date indicate that epirubicin appears to be at least comparable, and perhaps somewhat better than doxorubicin in clinical efficacy and is less cardiotoxic. Irreversible damage to heart muscle appears to occur in less than 1% of patients treated with epirubicin compared to a much higher rate with Adriamycin. However, there appears to be a risk of treatment-related leukemia in women receiving epirubicin.

- Taxanes (paclitaxel, docetaxel)

The Taxanes are a group of drugs that include paclitaxel (Taxol) and docetaxel (Taxotere) which are used in the treatment of breast and ovarian, as well as other, cancers.

Normally, microtubules are formed when a cell starts dividing and once the cell ceases to divide, microtubules are broken down and destroyed so the cell can function properly. These drugs act by blocking cell microtubules from breaking down so that cells become clogged with microtubules and cannot divide and grow.

Paclitaxel was FDA approved in 1992, and docetaxel in 1995, for the treatment of breast and ovarian cancer that recurs within 6 months after adjuvant chemotherapy, or has spread (metastasized) to nearby lymph nodes or other parts of the body.

Both of these drugs produce side effects that can be serious such as allergic reactions, bone marrow damage, anemia, and infection. Other disturbing side effects may include joint or muscle pain, diarrhea, nausea and vomiting, numbness and tingling, and loss of hair. Nevertheless, for many patients, the benefits of these drugs appear to outweigh the risk associated with use.

Clinical trials are in progress to evaluate the effectiveness of docetaxel alone, or in combination with other chemotherapeutic agents in the treatment of breast cancer.

- Biophosphonates (pamidronate, alendronate, zoledronic acid)

  Treatments discussed previously involve removing the cancer surgically and/or killing or controlling the cancer cells by a variety of means. Another approach is to alter the tissue environment in which metastatic cancer cells are growing.

Breast cancer metastasizes to bone causing an increase in resorption (breakdown), weaker bones, resulting fractures, and bone pain/discomfort.

Pamidronate (Aredia) is a biphosphonate drug that was FDA approved in 2001 for the treatment of bone metastases. Clinical studies have shown that women with bone metastases given pamidronate have decreased breakdown of bone, fewer new bone metastases, decreased bone fractures, and less bone pain and discomfort.

Zoledronic acid (Zometa) is another biphosphonate drug approved by the FDA in February, 2002, as useful for treating osteolytic effects and pain/discomfort from breast cancer bone metastases.

5.6   Hormonal therapy

Hormonal therapy is designed to keep cancer cells from obtaining the hormones in the body that they need to grow and spread.

- Tamoxifen (Nolvadex)

  Tamoxifen is an orally administered hormonal therapy that acts as an anti-estrogen, blocking the growth stimulating effects of the female hormone (estrogen) on breast cancer cells. It has been available now for over 20 years and found to be particularly useful as:
  - adjuvant, or additional, therapy following surgery and/or radiation treatment
  - treatment to reduce the chance of a woman at high risk developing breast cancer
  - an aid in preventing the spread, recurrence, and development of a new breast cancer in the other breast.

In the NCI Breast Cancer Prevention Trial (BCPT) tamoxifen was reported to produce approximately a 50% reduction in the: 1) occurrence of invasive breast cancer, and 2) diagnosis of non-invasive breast tumors such as ductal or lobular carcinoma in situ.

While the use of tamoxifen is reported to be largely beneficial, there are certain risks associated with the drug. Some of these risks are even life threatening. Therefore, one must carefully consider benefits versus risks before using the drug. Some of the more important increased serious risks include: 1) uterine cancer, 2) stroke, 3) blood clots, 4) cataracts, and 5) premature menopause. Nevertheless, it is generally believed that the benefits of tamoxifen as a treatment for breast cancer are now firmly established and far outweigh potential risks.

Patients with advanced breast cancer may take tamoxifen for varying periods of time depending on response and other factors. However, tamoxifen now is generally prescribed only for 5 years when used as adjuvant therapy for early stage breast cancer. As a treatment to reduce the chance of developing cancer in women at high risk, tamoxifen may be used for longer periods of time.

Young women at high risk are most likely to benefit from tamoxifen because their breast cancer risk substantially outweighs the potential for adverse effects. Also, women of any age without a uterus, who therefore are not at risk of endometrial cancer, may benefit accordingly. Older women have a higher risk of bone fractures that may be reduced by tamoxifen but these individuals are generally at higher risk for strokes and pulmonary embolisms which may be increased by tamoxifen. On the other hand, black women tend to have higher rates for strokes and pulmonary embolisms and lower rates of endometrial cancer, all of which may be increased by tamoxifen, and lower rates for hip fractures which tamoxifen helps prevent. Thus, the decision to take tamoxifen or not, depends on a number of factors, not just breast cancer risk.

Since the late 1980s, radiation and hormonal therapy (tamoxifen) have been given to women who had surgery for early breast cancer. These therapies were demonstrated to dramatically reduce the risk of cancer recurring. However, the question remained whether or not women with breast cancer needed to undergo the burden of both therapies and their side effects/complications. Results of a study in 1,000 women recently were presented at the 2000 Annual Meeting of the American Society of Clinical Oncology and answered the question rather clearly–that combination therapy remains the standard of care for most patients and tamoxifen cannot replace radiotherapy. Study results showed that after surgery and 5 years of treatment, the recurrence rate–or the proportion of women who had their cancer return in the same breast was 10.7% in the tamoxifen alone group, 4.8% in the radiotherapy alone group, and 2% in the combined (radiation plus tamoxifen) group. These results were interpreted to mean that standard care remains unchanged even for these very small, favorable tumors–one centimeter or smaller in size. This study also confirmed that tamoxifen also reduces the occurrence of contralateral breast cancer–the same disease in the other breast. The incidence of contralateral breast cancer was found to be 0.6% in the group given tamoxifen and 3% in the others.

• Aromatase Inhibitors (anastrozole, letrozole, exemestane)

While Tamoxifen has been well established as an effective hormonal therapy for a number of years, its use remains somewhat limited chiefly because of side effects. There is concern over a 2-7 times increase in uterine endometrial cancer in women who have taken the drug for over

5 years as well as significant increases in the incidence of stroke, pulmonary emboli, blood clots, cataracts, etc.

The search for more efficacious and safer agents has led to the development of a new class of drugs called aromatase inhibitors. Aromatase is an enzyme found in the adrenal glands, fat, muscle and breast tissue. The enzyme converts testosterone and androstendione into estrogen in the body. And studies have shown that this enzyme is responsible for most of the estrogen found in postmenopausal women.

Approximately two thirds of patients have hormone-dependent breast cancer containing estrogen receptors and requiring estrogen for growth. The vast majority of these patients have aromatase in their breast tissue providing the cancer with its own supply of estrogen.

Blocking aromatase with inhibitors has been shown to be an effective way of reducing estrogen levels in the breast and other parts of the body. Three such aromatase inhibitors are FDA approved for treating breast cancer, namely anastrozole, (Armidex), letrozcle (Femara), and exemestane (Aromasin).

Anastrozole (Armidex) was FDA approved in late 2000 for the treatment of postmenopausal women with hormone receptor positive or hormone receptor unknown locally advanced or metastatic breast cancer. The drug has been shown to be essentially comparable to tamoxifen in treating metastatic breast cancer. Clinical trials of anastrozole versus tamoxifen are in the process of being conducted to establish the role of anastrozole as first-line treatment of earlier stages of breast cancer. Results to date indicate that 5 years of adjuvant therapy with anastrozole may be better (by approximately 17%) in terms of disease-free survival compared to tamoxifen. Also, anastrozole therapy appears to be associated with significantly less contralateral new breast cancer (relative risk reduction of over 50%). Patients receiving anastrozole also appear to complain of less hot flashes, weight gain, vaginal bleeding and discharge, cerebrovascular and venous thrombosis and endometrial cancer than those receiving tamoxifen.

Letrozole (Femara) is another newer aromatase inhibitor which was FDA approved in early 2001 for first-line hormonal therapy in postmenopausal women with advanced estrogen receptor positive, or hormone receptor unknown, breast cancer. Available data on this drug also appears to indicate that it is superior to tamoxifen with regard to time to progression and objective clinical response rate. However, overall survival rates do not seem to differ significantly, except for possible superiority during the first 2 years of treatment. Patients with breast cancer progressing on tamoxifen also appear to benefit from letrozole therapy.

Exemestane (Aromasin) was FDA approved in late 1999 for the treatment of advanced breast cancer in postmenopausal women whose breast disease progressed following tamoxifen therapy. This drug is an irreversible steroidal aromatase inhibitor that also significantly lowers estrogen concentrations in the body. It has been shown to have clinical utility in the treatment of advanced breast.

In the coming years, the majority of breast cancer patients with hormone receptor positive tumors will have been exposed to adjuvant therapy with tamoxifen. At that time, one or more aromatase inhibitors may become first-line hormonal therapy in postmenopausal patients. Well-controlled comparative clinical trial data will be needed by then to decide which aromatase inhibitors to consider for use as replacement for tamoxifen.

Aromatase inhibitors appear to represent an important new class of hormonal agents for the management of breast cancer. They have more or less replaced earlier drugs used in advanced breast cancer. Better tolerability, increased potency and specificity, and clinical efficacy, have provided the rationale for using an aromatase inhibitor as adjuvant treatment of breast cancer in sequence, instead of, and in combination with tamoxifen. The emergence of estrogen as a mechanism for the development of breast cancer carcinogenesis provides additional rationale for considering aromatase inhibitors in the chemoprevention and treatment of breast cancer. Results of such trials will determine how widely aromatase inhibitors replace tamoxifen as first-line adjuvant therapy in breast cancer.

For additional information, consult FDA at http://www.fda.gov and/or NCI at http://www.cancer.gov.

5.7   Ovarian Ablation

Ovarian ablation by surgery or radiation has been shown to significantly improve the overall 15-year breast cancer survival rate in premenopausal women but not in those who are postmenopausal. In trials comparing ablation plus chemotherapy to chemotherapy alone, the benefit of ablation is seen only in the estrogen receptor positive subgroup.

The problem with surgical or radiation ovarian ablation approaches to improving breast cancer survival is that both procedures are irreversible. If they don't work, ovarian function cannot be restored and such women remain permanently menopausal.

Today, there are leuteinizing hormone-releasing hormone (LHRH), also known as gonadotropin-releasing hormone (GnRH) agonists, that block ovarian function and produce menopause. One of the drugs in this class that has been most tested for breast cancer survival is goserelin (Zoladex). It produces essentially the same hormonal effects as oophorectomy (surgical ablation) in terms of decreasing hormone production by the ovaries and its effects are considered to be "reversible". However, results from well-controlled clinical trials to establish reversibility and the efficacy and safety of gonadotropin-releasing hormone agonists in prolonging survival of breast cancer patients are not yet available. Further information regarding clinical trials of such agents may be obtained from the NCI at: http://www.cancer.gov.

5.8   Biological Therapy

The treatment of breast cancer has been focused primarily on surgery, radiation, chemotherapy and hormonal therapy. More recently biological therapies have been introduced as more is learned about how the body fights cancer on its own. Therapies that use the immune system to fight cancer are called biological therapies

- Herceptin Immunotherapy:

    Approximately 30% of women with metastatic breast cancer exhibit an overexpression (too many copies) of Her-2 neu oncogene that is reported to promote breast cancer growth and spread. Herceptin (trastuzumab) is a genetically engineered monocloncal antibody that blocks the breast cancer growth stimulating effects of this oncogene.

    Herceptin was FDA approved in September 1998 for the treatment of metastatic breast cancer with an overexpression of the Her-2 protein. The FDA also approved the DAKO Hercept Test in 1998 that is designed to measure levels of Her-2 protein in breast cancer tumor patients.

Clinical studies comparing Herceptin plus CT with CT alone have shown the Herceptin-treated patients experienced significantly longer median time to disease progression, higher overall response rate, longer median duration of response, and a higher one-year survival rate (80% in Herceptin group vs. 70% in the chemotherapy alone-treated patients).

Selection of patients who are considered likely to benefit from Herceptin is important because of serious risks in taking the drug (i.e., weakening of heart muscle leading to congestive heart failure in some patients, etc.). It is not known at this time if Herceptin has any beneficial effects in breast cancer patients with normal levels of Her-2 protein. Clinical studies are ongoing to establish the role of Herceptin in the treatment of earlier stages of breast cancer and its anti-angiogenesis (blocking of new blood vessel formation needed for cancer growth and spread) effects in the progression of the disease.

• Vaccine Therapy

Cancer vaccines are an emerging type of biological therapy. The FDA has not yet approved any cancer vaccine for use as standard treatment but a number are now being tested against a variety of cancer types including breast cancer.

Breast cancer vaccine research is still in the very early stages of development, and much work still needs to be done to show clear evidence of benefit. A number of approaches are currently under investigation and researchers still do not know if whole cell cancer vaccines or cancer antigen vaccines are best.

Currently, clinical trials testing certain breast cancer vaccines are underway. There are several places where patients can look for a possible trial in which to participate. Two such places include:

• NCI–Clinical Trials Database (PDQ)

Contains NCI-sponsored and drug company-sponsored trials. To access, go to the PDQ search form on the first search page and select the appropriate type of cancer (breast cancer) and on the second page, select "vaccine therapy" from the treatment modality list.

• NCI–Designated Cancer Center Web Sites

Search for breast cancer vaccine trials

Patients should be cautioned that if there is a standard treatment available to treat their breast cancer, they should not choose an experimental vaccine, unless standard therapy has failed. However, an experimental breast cancer vaccine may be considered as an appropriate addition to standard therapy, but not a replacement, under certain circumstances.

In animal studies, cancer vaccines appear to show the most potential promise in preventing cancer from recurring after the primary tumor has been eliminated by standard therapy. Treating existing new cancerous tumors with vaccines appears to be much more difficult. It remains to be established whether or not patients with breast cancer respond in a similar fashion.

5.9   Bone Marrow/Stem Cell Transplantations

Bone marrow is the soft, sponge-like material found inside bones which gives rise to the circulating red and white blood cells and platelets. It contains immature cells called stem cells that may be made to produce the entire range of mature circulating whole blood cells and other cells in the body depending on circumstances. Most of the body's stem cells are found in the bone marrow (BMSC) but some are peripheral blood stem cells (PBSC) found in the circulating blood stream. Umbilical cord blood also contains stem cells (UCBSC) that can divide to form more stem cells, or can mature into white or red blood cells, or platelets, the three main types of circulating whole blood cells.

Chemotherapy and radiation therapy can reduce the bone marrow's ability to make whole blood cells and cause anemia and the body's ability to fight infection. Bone marrow transplantation (BMT) and peripheral blood stem cell transplantation (PBSCT) are procedures that can restore stem cells and other blood cells that have been destroyed by high doses of chemotherapy and/or radiation therapy.

There are three main types of such transplants, namely:

- Autologous–patients receive their own stem cells
- Syngeneic–patients receive stem cells from their identical twin
- Allogeneic–patients receive closely matched stem cells from someone other than the patient or an identical twin, e.g., brother, sister, or parent–any of whom may serve as the donor–or an unrelated donor may be recruited

The main purpose of BMT and PBSCT in cancer treatment is to make it possible for patients to receive high doses of chemotherapy and/or radiation to conquer cancer and survive. However, as yet, BMT and PBSCT remain to be established as clinically useful in breast cancer treatment. Further information on BMT and PBSCT is available on line at http://www.cancer.gov via the NCI report entitled "Bone Marrow Transplantation and Peripheral Blood Stem Cell Transplantation: Questions and Answers".

Nevertheless, BMT and PBSCT clinical trials may be considered as a treatment option for select patients with advanced metastatic breast cancer that has not responded to standard treatment or in cases in which cancer has recurred. Further information concerning BMT and PBSCT clinical trials is available from the NCI on line at http://www.cancer.gov via a report entitled: "Taking Part in Clinical Trials: What Cancer Patients Need to Know".

5.10   Complementary and Alternative Medicine Therapies

Alternative therapies are ones that are used instead of mainstream or standard therapies of orthodox medicine in treatment. Whether any of these therapies has any anti-cancer utility remains to be established. A list of such therapies and their status in treatment may be obtained from the National Cancer Institute at http://www.cancer.gov or the FDA at: http://www.fda.gov.

Complementary therapies are ones meant chiefly to treat symptoms and improve quality of life. They are given in conjunction with mainstream or standard treatment largely as supportive care. Some are regarded in "certain circles" as having a "positive effect" on outcome but such remains to be confirmed in well-controlled clinical trials. Whether "positive effects" are the result of the patient's belief system, other factors, or the complementary therapy itself remains to be demonstrated. Complementary therapies may include such approaches as:

- Acupuncture
- Bioelectric/magnetic
- Counseling
- Diet/nutrition
- Herbs
- Homeopathy

- Massage
- Meditation
- Prayer
- Psychic healing
- Support groups
- Therapeutic touch
- Visualization/imagery
- Vitamins/minerals

Further information/reports on complementary and alternative medicine therapies, may be obtained from the National Center for Complementary and Alternative Medicine at http://www.nccam.nih.gov. National Cancer Institute reports on such approaches may be reviewed online at http://www.cancer.gov via the following:

- "Questions and answers about complementary and alternative medicine in cancer treatment"
- "Levels of evidence for human studies of cancer complementary and alternative medicine"

5.11 Treatment Options

Treatment options vary according to the stage and type of breast cancer, among other factors.

Stage 0, carcinoma in situ, options may include observation alone, lumpectomy alone, or lumpectomy plus radiation. Outlook generally is considered to be excellent and almost all such patients survive for many years. In fact, the vast majority of such patients may be considered "cured" after appropriate therapy.

Stages I-III treatment options include more aggressive approaches such as lumpectomy or mastectomy plus radiotherapy, chemotherapy, and hormonal therapy (in estrogen receptor positive tumors). Outlook generally is good for most stage II tumors with 75-90% surviving for 5-10 years and longer. In Stage III, the outlook becomes less favorable with only 50% or so of patients surviving 5 years or beyond. Herceptin may be added to Her-2 positive tumor patients in stage IV, and perhaps even in earlier stages, to improve outlook. However, 5-year survival for all stage IV patients is only around 15-20%.

A 3-tiered TNM risk classification for patients with breast cancer and negative axillary lymph nodes has been devised by an international consensus panel. TNM is based on tumor size, estrogen or progesterone receptor status, and tumor grade and is believed to help improve choice of therapy and resulting outcome.

Risk is classified in this system as follows:

Table I Risk Classification: Negative Axillary Nodes

Criteria Graded	Low Risk	Intermediate Risk	High Risk
Tumor size	<1–1 cm*	1–2 cm	> 2 cm
Receptor status**	Positive	Positive	Negative
Tumor grade	G I	G I–II	G II–III

* = centimeters
** = estrogen or progesterone
G = tumor grade class I–III

The higher the risk, the more aggressive the therapy needed and the poorer the outlook in general. However, certain tumors with uncommon histologies (mucinous, medullary carcinomas) also have a favorable prognosis and are considered to be low risk. The level of Her-2 receptor protein and tumor cell proliferation (S-phase fraction) and ploidy also are believed to be useful markers in defining risk of lymph node-negative disease, treatment and outcome.

CT and hormonal regimens appear to offer about the same basic benefit to patients regardless of whether their axillary lymph nodes are positive or negative. As a result, adjuvant therapy is based largely on assessment of the risk of tumor recurrence versus the short and long term risks of adjuvant therapy, and is tailored to the patient's particular set of circumstances. Based on these considerations, among others, adjuvant treatment options may include the following:

Table II Adjuvant Treatment Options: Lymph Node Negative Patients

Patient Group	Low Risk	Intermediate Risk	High Risk
PM, ER(–) or PR(+)	None or TAM alone	TAM alone	CT + TAM, or CT +OA, or CT + TAM + OA
PM, ER(–) Or PR (–)	NA	NA	CT
Post-M, ER(–) or PR(+)	None or TAM alone	TAM +CT, or TAM alone	TAM + CT, or TAM alone

Table III Treatment Options: Lymph Node Positive Patients

Patient Group	Treatment Options
PM, ER(–) or PR(–)	CT + TAM, or CT + OA, or CT +TAM + OA
PM, ER(–) or PR(–)	CT
Post-M, ER(–) or PR(+)	TAM + CT, or TAM alone
Post-M, ER(–) or PR(–)	CT
>70 years of age	TAM alone, or CT if receptor negative

Legend for Tables II and III

PM = premenopausal   TAM = tamoxifen
Post-M = postmenopausal   CT = chemotherapy
ER = estrogen receptor   OA = ovarian ablation
PR = progesterone receptor   NA = information not available
(–) = negative
(+) = positive

Consensus opinion regarding treatment options indicates that:

- Treatment with a combination of chemotherapy drugs improves survival and probably should be given to most pre- and post-menopausal women with localized breast cancer regardless of lymph node involvement or estrogen receptor status
- Including one of the anthracycline drugs as part of the chemotherapy regiment produces a small but statistically significant survival advantage
- Hormonal therapy benefits women whose cancers have estrogen receptors regardless of age, menopausal status, tumor size, or whether the cancer has spread to nearby lymph nodes

- Five years of hormonal therapy now remains the standard with tamoxifen
- Women who have had mastectomies and who are at high risk for recurrence of cancer, women who have undergone mastectomy and who have four or more cancerous lymph nodes, or advanced primary tumor benefit most from post surgical radiotherapy

Additional information on treatment options may be obtained from the NCI report entitled: "Breast Cancer (PDQ): Treatment" available online at http://www.cancer.gov.

5.12   Treatment Updates

- Updates

  Recent NCI Breast Cancer Updates/Reports are available online at http://www.cancer.gov on the following topics, among others:
  - Tamoxifen lowers risk of benign breast disease
  - Breast cancer trials continue to show no benefit from high dose CT with stem cell transplantation, no advantage over intermediate-dose CT alone
  - Herceptin improves treatment of metastatic breast cancer
  - Way to treat very small tumors—post surgical adjuvant therapy should be considered an option
  - Tamoxifen doesn't prevent heart disease on short-term treatment
  - CT with an appropriate combination regimen improves survival and is recommended for most women with localized disease
  - Sentinel node biopsy trials underway to evaluate the pros and cons of the procedure
  - Herceptin clinical trials in non-metastic breast cancer

- Tamoxifen found to be equally effective in black and white women
- Radiation plus tamoxifen reduces breast cancer recurrence
- Early breast cancer patients benefit from shortened chemotherapy
- Breast cancer prevention trial ongoing
- Tamoxifen versus raloxifene comparison (STAR trial status report)
- Raloxifene (Evista) trial to prevent breast cancer in women at high risk
- Tamoxifen—5 years is enough to prevent relapse/recurrence
- Tamoxifen prevention trial - approximately 50% reduction in breast cancer
- Digital mammography trial update
- Core needle breast biopsy is reported to be an accurate alternative to surgical excision

- Overall Prognosis/Survival Statistics

  The clinical stage of breast cancer at the time of diagnosis appears to be a reasonably good indicator for prognosis (probable treatment outcome) and survival. A number of additional factors besides staging can influence the recommended treatment and likely outcome in any given patient. Some of these factors may include: tumor appearance, precise cell type, aggressive features of the cancer, presence or absence of certain biomarkers, and TNM classification, among others.

  Overall 5- year survival rates for patients treated according to the stage of the disease are considered to be approximately as follows:

Stage of Breast Cancer and Survival

Stage	5-Year Survival or Better
0	95-100%
I	90-95%
II	75-85%
III	50-60%
IV	15-20%

Involvement of axillary lymph nodes adversely affects prognosis/survival.

CT and hormone therapy improves prognosis for most patients and increases the likelihood of improved survival in those with stages I-III breast cancer.

CHAPTER 6

Coping with Cancer

Following a diagnosis of cancer and/or treatment, patients often become overwhelmed with new information/issues, and the need to accept unwelcomed alternatives or change. They need to learn how to cope with their cancer, treatment, complications, side effects and other important issues. Coping may be facilitated through various support groups/organizations, information, and therapy.

6.1   Support Groups

Support for coping is available in a number of different ways according to the issue(s) at hand. Reports on ways to cope are available online from the National Cancer Institute at: http://www.cancer.gov, and include:

- General Support Information

  - Questions and Answers About the Cancer Information Service
  - Facing Forward: A Guide for Cancer Survivors
  - How to Find Resources in Your Own Community If You Have Cancer
  - Support for People With Cancer and the People Who Care for Them
  - When Cancer Recurs: Meeting the Challenge

- When Someone in Your Family Has Cancer
- Your Health Care Team: Your Doctor is Only the Beginning

- Support Organizations

  - Questions and Answers About Finding Cancer Support Groups
  - National Organizations That Offer Services to People With Cancer and Their Families

- Supportive Expressive Group Therapy (SEGT)

  SEGT professional counseling is available for those with life-threatening illnesses. It encourages participants to express feelings and concerns about their illness and its effects on their lives in the supported environment of a therapist-led group. SEGT does not prolong survival in women with breast cancer but it is reported to improve pain control, mood, and quality of life. For additional information, see the following recently published articles on the subject:

  - "The Effect of Group Psychosocial Support on Survival in Metastatic Breast Cancer" by Goodwin, P.J. et al, *The New England Journal of Medicine*, 245(24): 1719-1726, December 13, 2001.
  - "Mind Matter–Group Therapy and Survival in Breast Cancer" by Spiegel, D., *The New England Journal of Medicine*, 245(24): 1767-1768, December 13, 2001.

6.2   Side Effects/Complications

A number of reports on side effects, complications, and remedies are available online from the NCI at http://www.cancer.gov. These include information on side effects and complications such as:

- Anxiety
- Constipation, fecal impaction, bowel obstruction
- Delirium, confused thinking
- Depression
- Fatigue
- Fever, chills, sweats
- Hair loss
- Hypercalcemia (high blood calcium)
- Lymphedema
- Loss, grief, bereavement
- Premature menopause, hot flashes, etc.
- Mouth sores/ulcers, dryness, bleeding gums
- Nausea, vomiting
- Nutritional issues
- Post traumatic stress disorders
- Pruritis
- Radiation enteritis
- Sexual and reproductive issues
- Sleep disorders (insomnia, disturbed sleep cycle)
- Substance abuse
- Superior vena cava syndrome

These reports as well as others may help patients to better understand and cope with such side effects/complications.

6.3   Treatment Related Issues

- Chemotherapy and You: A Guide to Self-Help During Cancer Treatment
- Helping Yourself During Chemotherapy
- A New Treatment for Hot Flashes: Antidepressants
- Radiation Therapy and You: A Guide to Self-Help During Cancer Treatment
- Smoking Cessation and Continued Risk in Cancer Patients

6.4   Hospice, Home Care, Health Care

- Hospice
- Home Care For Cancer Patients
- Advanced Cancer: Living Each Day
- Loss, Grief and Bereavement (PDQ)
- Transitional Care Planning (PDQ)

6.5   End-of-Life Issues

- Advanced Directives
- Advanced Cancer: Living Each Day
- Loss, Grief and Bereavement

CHAPTER 7

Clinical Trials

Clinical trials may be a useful "treatment" alternative for selected patients with breast cancer.

Information on NCI clinical trials is available at http://www.cancer.gov. Click on "Clinical Trials' site and then on to "Breast Cancer" or "Search NCI Clinical Trials" sites.

Within the 'Clinical Trials' site reports are provided on:
- Finding Ways to Look for Specific Cancer Trials
- Trial Information Grouped by Type of Cancer
- Understanding What Clinical Trials Are and How they Work
  - Clinical Trials Explained
  - Participant Protection
- Recent developments in new clinical trials reports include:
  - New Treatments
  - Prevention
  - Testing and Screening
  - Patient Care Costs
- Clinical Trial Results

- Resources for patients and healthcare professionals

The "Understanding Clinical Trials" site provides information/reports on:
- What is a Clinical Trial
- Should I Take Part in a Clinical Trial
- How do I Take Part in a Clinical Trial
- Participating in a Trial: Questions to Ask You Doctor
- Q and A: Access to Investigational Drugs
- How is a Clinical Trial Planned and Carried out
- Clinical Trials and Insurance Coverage: A Resource Guide
- Understanding the Approval process of New Cancer Drugs
- Facts and Figures About Cancer Clinical Trials
- Ten things to Know About Cancer Treatment Trials
- Taking Part in Clinical Trials: What Cancer Patients Need to Know

Patients may benefit from clinical trials of promising new experimental treatments that are not yet FDA approved. Bear in mind that clinical trials of new therapies are the principle way advances in treatment are made. Thus, a clinical trial of an experimental therapy may be worthwhile to consider under certain circumstances.

Most treatment cancer trials are designed to compare a new experimental treatment with a standard treatment employing random assignment of patients to each group. While some patients may receive a placebo in clinical trials, use of placebos in cancer treatment trials is rare today. Also, bear in mind that experimental treatments under study are not always better than, or even as good as, available standard care, and they may even produce unexpected serious side effects.

Before taking part in a clinical trial, patients should seriously consider all the pros and cons regarding participation from a patient's point of view. The NCI report entitled "Taking Part in Clinical Trials; What Cancer Patients Need to Know", available on line at http://www.cancer.gov, provides information on issues patients need to think about and understand fully beforehand.

Also, one needs to consider that healthcare plans and managed care providers do not always cover all patient care costs involved in a clinical trial. In this regard, patients should read the NCI report available at: http://www.cancer.gov entitled: "Clinical Trials and Insurance Coverage: A Resource Guide".

CHAPTER 8

Male Breast Cancer

Less than 1% of all breast cancer occurs in men. Compared to female, male breast cancer is considered to be rare. While men of all ages may be affected, the mean age for diagnosis of breast cancer in males is between 60 and 70.

Several factors are reported to increase the risk of male breast cancer. These may include:

- Diseases associated with hyperestrogenism such as cirrhosis of the liver or Klinefelter's syndrome
- Estrogen administration
- Familial tendencies such as female relatives with breast cancer
- Genetic factors such as BRCA-2 or other gene mutations

Male breast tumor pathology is similar to female breast cancer. Infiltrating ductual carcinoma is the most common form encountered. Paget's disease of the nipple and ductal carcinoma in situ also occur but lobular carcinoma in situ has not been described to date.

TNM staging and spread of male breast cancer is similar to that seen in females.

Treatment options may include:

- Modified radical mastectomy with axillary dissection and radiation
- Adjuvant therapy on the same basis as for women
- Chemotherapy plus tamoxifen and other hormonal therapy—in node positive patients. Approximately 85% of all male breast cancers are estrogen receptor positive and 70% progesterone receptor positive, and the presence of receptors correlates with response to hormone therapy.
- Chemotherapy usually includes:
  - CMF (cyclophosphamide, methotrexate, 5-fluorouracil), or
  - CAM (cyclophosphamide, Adriamyicn, 5-fluorouracil)
- Tamoxifen use is associated with a high rate of treatment limiting side effects in a significant number of patients
- Surgical excision or radiation therapy combined with chemotherapy is usually used for locally recurrent disease.

Prognostic factors and survival are similar in male breast cancer compared to women with comparable disease.

Treatment modalities may include:

- Aminoglutethimide
- Aromatase inhibitors for estrogen receptor-positive patients
- Chemotherapy
- Leutenizing hormone-releasing hormone agonist with or without androgen blockage (antiandrogen)
- Orchiectomy
- Progesterone
- Tamoxifen for estrogen receptor-positive patients

Hormonal modalities may be used sequentially. Chemotherapy with CMF or CAF usually are used after failure of hormonal therapy. Response with both hormonal and chemotherapy are similar to those seen in women with breast cancer. Metastases usually are treated with hormonal therapy, chemotherapy or a combination of both. Hormonal therapy may be used initially.

Additional information on male breast cancer is available from the following Web Resources:

- Harvard Medical School–http://www.hms.harvard.edu
- Mayo Clinic–http://www.mayo.edu
- National Cancer Institute–http://www.cancer.gov
- NOAH: New York Online Access to Health–http://www.noah-health.org
- Oncolink-University of Pennsylvania Cancer Center–http://www.oncolink.org

CHAPTER 9

Searching the Web

You are now in a position to ask all your questions and obtain desired answers from the Web about breast cancer. Many books have been written on how to use the Internet/Web. You can obtain one of your choice from your local public library, if you don't already have one, and use it accordingly.

A number of commercial services such as AOL, MSN, Netscape, Yahoo and others provide easy, reliable, and relatively inexpensive access to the Internet/Web via your computer. If you do not have a computer, you can use one at your local public, college or university library, and connect to the Internet/Web at no cost to you. And your local reference librarian can show you not only how to connect to the Web but also instruct you on how to use it properly to facilitate your search. Should a computer not be available, or if you prefer, you can use a WebTV or similar device hooked up to your TV set at home to connect to, and use, the Internet/Web. Once connected, you are ready to start searching using the Author's List of Useful Web Resources provided in Chapter 10. These are arranged alphabetically for ease of reference.

Not all breast cancer information made available on the Web should be considered current, comprehensive, and useful (CCU). Therefore, you are cautioned to be selective and use due diligence in your search. A good way to select useful Web Resources is to use reliable guidelines in choosing them. Such guidelines may be obtained from a number of sources such as:

- American Medical Association–http://www.ama-assn.org/about-guide-lines.htm
- Healthfinder–http://www.healthfinder.gov
- Health on the Net Foundation - http://www.hon.ch

Criteria used by different organizations in selecting CCU Web resources varies. Nevertheless, using the guidelines developed by one or more of these organization should enable you to find the best Web Resources available for your purposes.

The Author's List of Useful Web Resources in Chapter 10 is a selection which, in the author's opinion, provide CCU information for the vast majority of those consumers, health care providers, patients, and physicians who may use this book.

The Web is currently estimated at well over 2 billion pages and 3 billion documents, and is still growing rapidly each day. When you search the Web with a search engine such as Google.com, etc., you are not searching it directly as this is not possible at this time. The Web is the totality of all the Web pages and documents that reside on computers (called servers), worldwide, and your computer cannot locate or search them directly. All you can do with your computer is to go to one of a number of intermediate resources that contain selected and organized Web pages and databases. Thus, you merely search these intermediate resources and they provide you with links to the Web page needed to complete your search. You then can click on these Web pages/links and retrieve documents/information pertaining to your search.

Google.com can provide you with a reasonably complete search of the entire Web, usually in less than a second or so. However, then you are left with the very difficult task of reviewing all the Web pages/documents discovered to find the one(s) that meet your CCU needs. This not only would be time consuming, but also well beyond the capability, for most people to do in a reasonable period of time.

To simplify matters, the author has personally selected and assembled a list of 60 key Web Resources that provide what may be considered to be CCU information. These are listed alphabetically for ease of reference for you in Chapter 10. The main content of each of these Web Resources has been organized into categories and topics in such a way as to facilitate your selection of the one(s) that are most likely to provide you with the particular information you need.

For a general or a specific topic search, a good place to start your selection of appropriate Web Resources includes one or more of the 5 Web Resources listed below from the Author's List in Chapter 10. These are:

- Healthfinder - http://www.healthfinder.gov
- Medlineplus–http://nlm.nih.gov/medlineplus
- National Cancer Institute–http://www.cancer.gov
- NOAH: New York Online Access to Health–http://www.noah-health.org
- PubMed–http://www.ncbi.nlm.nih.gov/PubMed

The author's two favorite Web Resources as a starting point for most searches are:

- National Cancer Institute
- PubMed

Information is provided both in English and Spanish by both.

The National Cancer Institute is regarded as the single best Web Resource for one to initiate a search for CCU breast cancer information.

The 5 Web Resources cited above provide information at different levels of complexity for consumers, healthcare providers, patients, and physicians, alike. Choose the one(s) most appropriate for your needs.

Medical colleges and university hospital medical centers also provide CCU information. Ones to consider include:

- Harvard Medical School–http://www.hms.harvard.edu
- Mayo Clinic–http://www.mayo.edu
- Oncolink–University of Pennsylvania Cancer Center–http://www.oncolink.org
- University of Wisconsin Comprehensive Cancer Center–http://www.wisc.edu

The author's two preferences from this group are:

- Harvard Medical School
- Oncolink–University of Pennsylvania Cancer Center

You may use these or others as you deem appropriate for your needs from the Author's List in Chapter 10.

The Komen Breast Center Foundation (http:www.komen.org) is the author's preference regarding a public non-profit foundation providing CCU information.

Health on the Net Foundation (http://www.hon.ch) located in Geneva, Switzerland is one of the best international Web Resources available and should be considered in any search. This site offers CCU information for consumers, healthcare providers, patients, and physicians in a number of foreign languages of your choice.

NOAH: New York Online Access to Health (http://www.noah-health.org) is a highly regarded Web Resource providing CCU information for both patients and healthcare professionals. Information is provided in English and Spanish.

Information for all 60 Web Resources is organized by topics/categories to simplify selection by you and expedite your search. In the event you cannot easily find a Web Resource that contains the category(s)/topic(s) of information you are looking for, you can use the search site on one or more of the U.S. Government or medical college or university medical center Web Resources to search for and obtain desired information.

Remember that the Web is growing rapidly and, as a result, is in a constant state of flux and reorganization. Web Resources may change their names and/or Web addresses, formats, scope and categorization of information offered, and more. If for any reason the Website address you choose from the Author's List doesn't work when you try to connect, search the Web Resource name. If you still have problems connecting, try another Search Engine or an alternative Web Resource from the Author's List.

Keep in mind that various Web Resources use different methods to search the Web to compile their databases and information offered. Also, each organizes and categorizes information differently, some better than others. Thus, searches likely may provide results that differ and need to be reconciled.

For the most part, information you find via the Author's List of Useful Web Resources likely will be reasonably useful in most respects but not necessarily all. Thus, you should not necessarily believe all information you obtain from any one Web Resource. Unlike scientific articles published in peer reviewed professional journals, there is no guarantee that the information you obtain from any one Web Resource will be CCU. Also, keep in mind that not all Web Resources are uniformly reliable in all aspects of all information offered. Therefore, it is suggested that you select the most appropriate Web Resources for your purposes and compare and contrast the information obtained from at least 2-3 or more different ones before reaching any conclusions/decisions with your physician/healthcare provider. Even in the world of the Web, a second and even a third opinion is worthwhile.

One also needs to consider that even in the case of evidence-based information from well-controlled clinical trials, there are problems in terms of what the data collected mean. Evidence necessarily is subject to interpretation and application and these are subjective processes. All of us are biased to some degree in one way or another not only in obtaining, but also in interpreting and applying information, evidence-based or not. Word, phrases, statistics, etc. mean different things to different people depending on "where one is coming from". For example, even in the case of a long-standing document such as the Constitution of the United States, written by great minds some time ago—people, lawyers, judges, and even the Supreme Court still argue about, and have great difficulty interpreting and applying the "original intent" of our founding fathers who authored it.

Finally, you should note that not all treatments advocated at any time will necessarily be as useful as claimed. The history of breast cancer is replete with examples of past treatments, advocated by the leading figures of the time, that proved not to be very useful after all.

Nevertheless, available evidence indicates that vast improvements have been made in the diagnosis and treatment of breast cancer in the last 20-30 years. Breast cancer now can be successfully treated in the vast majority of cases and survival is constantly improving. New advances are being made every year and the future looks bright–so keep the faith–it is more important than you may think.

Recommended Further Readings

1. *Mammography and Beyond: Developing Technologies for the Early Detection of Breast Cancer*, Institute of Medicine and the National Research Council, edited by Nass, S.J., Henders, I.C., and Lashoff, J.C., National Academy Press, Washington, DC, 2001.

2. *Susan Love's Breast Book* by Susan M. Love, M. D., and Karen Lindsey, 3rd edition, Perseus Publishing, Cambridge, Massachusetts, 2000.

3. *The Breast Cancer Wars: Hope, Fear and the Pursuit of a Cure in Twentieth Century America* by Barron Lerner, M.D., Oxford University Press, New York, NY, 2001.

CHAPTER 10

Author's List of Useful Web Resources

10.1 **Alpha Cancer Information Resource**
http://www.alphacancer.com

Alpha Cancer Information Resource (ACIR) was formed in November 1997. It combines common interests and initiatives among the NCI sponsored Cancer Clinical Trials Cooperative Groups. It provides a unique opportunity for access to cancer-related health information on the Internet/Web and to interact directly with leading specialists in the field of breast cancer. Click on "breast cancer" for information of interest. Sites are featured for information on:

- Adjuvant therapy
- Clinical trials
- Complementary/alternative medicine approaches
- Detection
- Diagnoses
- Exercise connection
- Feature articles
- Genetics
- Herceptin
- New developments/latest advances in treatment

- New medications to reduce risk
- Patient advocacy
- Post-operative management guidelines
- Psychological issues/coping
- Reconstructive surgery
- Risk factors
- Sentinel node biopsy
- Side effects of chemotherapy management
- Screening, new techniques
  - Digital mammography
  - MRI (magnetic resonance imaging)
  - PET (positron emission tomography)
  - Ultrasound
- Treatment, management, latest advances
- Webcasts–experts in the field

Use Search site provided for additional information of interest.

10.2   American Academy of Family Physicians
http://www.aafp.org

The American Academy of Family Physicians (AAFP), founded in 1947, is the national association of family doctors with more than 93,000 members in the United States, Puerto Rico, the Virgin Islands and Guam. It promotes and maintains high quality standards for family doctors who are providing continuing comprehensive health care to the public.

AAFP provides useful breast cancer information from authoritative family physicians.

Use "Quick Search" site for information on specific topics of interest. Search "breast cancer", and click on topic of interest such as:

- Breast cancer diagnosis and screening
- Editorials on screening for breast cancer
- Evaluation of common breast problems
- Screening for genetic risk of breast cancer
- Other topics of interest

10.3   AMC Cancer Research Center
http://www.amc.org

AMC Cancer Research Center is a non-profit research institute dedicated to the prevention of cancer founded in 1989.

For available information on breast cancer go to "Cancer & Health Info" and clink on "Breast".

AMC states that 1 in 9 American women will develop breast cancer in their lifetime. Over 200,000 women in the United States are diagnosed with breast cancer every year and over 40,000 women will die annually from the disease. The earlier breast cancer is detected, the easier it is to treat. If detected early, before cancer cells have spread, the "cure rate" from breast cancer may be as high as 90% or even higher.

Patients should be active in early detection and prevention of breast cancer by: 1) conducting personal self-examinations each month; 2) having yearly clinical breast examinations by your doctor; 3) having a mammogram at age 40 and every 1-2 years thereafter; 4) adopting a diet low in fat; 5) being on the look out for lumps, changes in breast shape, pain or discharge from the nipples, and consulting your doctor if there are any questions or concerns.

10.4   American Cancer Society
http://www.cancer.org

The American Cancer Society (ACS) is a nationwide community-based voluntary health organization with state divisions and more than 3,400 local offices. It provides the latest breast cancer research news via:

- ACS News Today
- News Room

Click on "Health Information Seekers" and get facts on breast cancer, risk factors and prevention.

Use ACS Search site for more specific information on topics of interest. Your search for "breast cancer" information will yield information on topics such as:

- Drug guide
- Glossary
- News today
- Resource for ACS supporters
- Resources for health information seekers
- Resources for patients, family, friends and survivors

Use Advanced Search site for additional information.

10.5   American College of Obstetricians and Gynecologists
http://www.acog.org

The American College of Obstetricians and Gynecologists (ACOG), founded in 1951, has well over 40,000 members. It is regarded as one of the nation's leading group of board certified physicians providing health care information for women.

You may use the "Search the Public Web Site" for desired information on topics of interest.

Information provided is rated in percentages (i.e. 100% or less) as to how well it may conform to the topic/aspect searched

For example, in searching "breast cancer" the following information is made available and ranked. For details, you may click on the topics of interest:

- 25 years of research does not support the hypothesis that estrogen use increases the risk of breast cancer

- Articles in the Journal of the American Medical Association and the Journal of the National Cancer Institute report a modestly increased risk for breast cancer among women using estrogen-progestin combination hormone replacement therapy compared to women using estrogen only

- The vast majority of women with breast cancer (i.e. >90%) have no known risk factors for breast cancer.

- Only an estimated 5-7% of breast cancer cases appear to be linked to inherited mutations in genes known as BRCA-1 and BRCA-2.

- Breast feeding or trauma to the breast does not appear to lead to breast cancer.

- Have your obstetrician-gynecologist/physician examine your breasts to detect an abnormality you may have missed. If at high risk or if benign cysts make your breasts difficult to examine, more frequent exams may be a good idea. Mammograms detect breast lumps that are too small for you or your physician to feel.

- The Encyclopedia of Women's Health and Wellness, ACOG's database information is compiled and expanded to provide best advice for patients in one source. Consult this publication for breast self-exam information.

10.6   American College of Radiology
http://www.acr.org

The American College of Radiology (ACR), a non-profit professional society 30,000 members strong, is the principal organization of radiologists, radiation oncologists and clinical medical physicists in the United States. Its primary purposes are to improve service to the patient, advance the science of radiology, study the socioeconomic aspects of the practice of radiology and encourage continuing education for members.

The ACR, the American Cancer Society, the American Medical Women's Association and numerous national women's groups support annual mammography screening beginning by age 40. These groups also recommend at least yearly clinical breast examinations starting at age 40.

The ACR believes that clinical trials have shown that by having screening mammograms every year, compared to every 1-2 years as was recommended in the past for women in their 40s, breast cancers are found at an earlier stage and that the earlier breast cancers are detected, the better the changes for improved treatment results.

Sites are provided for pertinent information on:

- Accredited mammography facilities near you
- Breast care guidelines
- Mammography
- Medline (free access), National Library of Medicine, for search on topics of interest
- News
- Patient care

10.7 American Institute for Cancer Research
http://www.aicr.org

The American Institute for Cancer Research (ACIR) is a pioneer in the area of research related to diet and nutrition in the prevention and treatment of cancer. It serves as one of the USA's leading sources for educational programs for cancer prevention.

Scientific evidence suggests that a number of cancers may be preventable. This is beginning to have an effect as seen by the change being reported in dietary habits and in the reduction in a number of cancer rates that are now beginning to be observed. Further information is available on the links:

- Breast cancer video in English or Spanish
- Free booklets on breast cancer prevention
- Guidelines for lower cancer risk
- Information for cancer patients
- New free brochure offers fiber information
- Recent AICR press (news) updates
- Science advisory–researchers see obesity cancer link
- Stopping cancer before it starts

10.8   American Medical Association
http://www.ama-assn.org

The American Medical Association (AMA), founded more than 150 years ago, is regarded as the nation's leader in promoting professionalism in medicine. AMA's work includes the development and promotion of standards in medical practice, research, and education, and advocacy in behalf of patients and physicians. The AMA strives to serve as the voice of the American medical profession.

For information, click on "health professionals" or "patients" and use the Search site to obtain desired information on breast cancer topics of interest. Learn how to improve your health with easy-to-understand, high quality health information.

10.9   American Medical Women's Association
http://www.amwa-doc.org

The American Medical Women's Association (AMWA), an organization of over 10,000 women physicians and medical students, is dedicated to the care of the woman patient and her healthcare needs.

AMWA regards breast cancer as the second leading cause of death of women in the United States with approximately 200,000 new cases diagnosed annually.

AMWA Search site is provided to obtain information on topics of interest. This site is sponsored by:

- Cancer Treatment Centers–a comprehensive whole person approach to cancer treatment

- Emerging Med Cancer Patient Referral Service–free clinical trials matching and referral service for cancer patients using an up-to-date database of public and private cancer clinical trials. You are invited to find out if any of these trials are right for you.

Search "breast cancer" provides useful information on: 1) methods of early detection/screening, 2) risk factors, 3) diagnoses, 4) types of cancer, 5) treatment, 6) future of cancer research, 7) cancer care, 8) education for primary care providers/patients, and more.

10.10   American Pain Foundation
http://www.painfoundation.org

The American Pain Foundation (APF), founded in 1997, is an online resource center for people with pain, their families and caregivers. It is an independent non-profit organization serving people with pain through information, education, and advocacy. APF is dedicated to improving the quality of life for people with pain.

Sites are provided for information on:
* Advocacy
* Finding help
* Links for additional information
* News
* Pain action guide
* Pain care bill of rights
* Patient information and surveys
* Search site for more information on pain

10.11 American Society of Clinical Oncology
http://www.asco.org

The American Society of Clinical Oncology (ASCO), founded in 1964, has more than 16,000 professional members worldwide. ASCO provides a range of professionally edited information for oncology professionals and patients.

Information is provided on topics such as:

- Bilateral breast cancer
- Bone mineral density and risk of breast cancer
- BRCA1 and BRCA2 mutations and breast cancer
- Breast cancer surveillance guidelines
- Breast conservation therapy for familial breast cancer
- Breast conservation therapy for invasive breast cancer
- Breast magnetic resonance imaging and clinical management
- Breast size and local and distant recurrence
- Cancer health policy
- Cancer news
- Clinical research on breast cancer
- Conservative surgery and radiation therapy
- Detection of breast cancer cells in ductal lavage fluid
- FDA approves tamoxifen to reduce risk of breast cancer
- Feature articles
- First line treatment of advanced breast cancer
- Impact of national screening program
- Male breast cancer
- Male to female ratio for breast cancer

- Mammography
- People living with cancer
- Polychemotherapy for early breast cancer
- Primary chemotherapy can spare breasts
- Prophylactic mastectomy
- Results of post-operative radiotherapy
- Risks and benefits of tamoxifen and raloxifene
- Surgical management of breast cancer

A Search site is provided to obtain additional information.

10.12 American Society of Plastic Surgeons
http://www.plasticsurgery.org

The American Society of Plastic Surgeons (ASPS) and the Plastic Surgery Educational Foundation (PSEF) provide information on a wide variety of cosmetic and reconstructive plastic surgery procedures as well as offering a Plastic Surgeon Referral Service.

Sites are available for information on:
- Find a plastic surgeon
- Frequently asked questions and answers
- Medem which offers an extensive medical library for the public
- Medical professionals
- Patient advocacy
- Statistics and costs
- Surgical procedures

Using the ASPS search site for "breast reconstruction" provides information on:

- Center for Plastic Surgery–obtain an introductory look at the options available to women after a mastectomy
- E-sthetics–breast reconstruction–a plastic surgeon gives a brief summary of the operation to reconstruct the breast after a mastectomy
- Mastectomy and breast reconstruction–outlines the benefits of performing a breast reconstruction in conjunction with a mastectomy
- Olson Center for Women's Health–proper breast reconstruction is inherent to a woman's emotional recovery
- Patient advocate–support network to increase awareness of the options women have for breast reconstruction. Explore a topic or join a support group.
- PSIS–a copy of the 1998 Federal Breast Construction Law provided by the Plastic Surgery Information Service

10.13 Association of Cancer Online Resources
http://www.acor.org/index.html

The Association of Cancer Online Resources (ACOR) is a collection of cancer-related Web Resources that allow the patients/healthcare providers to find and use credible information relevant to breast cancer.

ACOR cancer information system currently offers access to electronic mailing lists and a variety of unique web sites. Mailing lists are specifically designed to be public online support groups providing information and community to thousands of patients, caregivers, or anyone looking for answers.

Sites are provided for:
- Cancer Net

- Chat
- Glossary
- Links
- Mailing lists

New sites include:
- Breast Cancer Support Group
- Current Advances in Breast Cancer Treatments

A Search site allows one to search the National Cancer Institute (NCI) databases. Included are the Breast Cancer Program Review Group Reports on:
- Biology–improving breast cancer diagnoses and treatment
- Control–improvements in breast cancer mortality
- Etiology–causes
- Executive summary
- Genetic testing–5-40% with altered BRCA1 gene and 10-20% with altered BRCA2 gene are expected to develop breast cancer.
- NCI initiatives
- Outcomes–tumor response, disease-free survival, overall survival
- Prevention studies
- Research
- *What You Need to Know*–NCI publication

10.14 Blood and Marrow Transplant Information Network
http://www.bmtnews.org

The Blood and Marrow Transplant Information Network (BMTIN), founded in 1990, is a non-profit organization dedicated exclusively to serving the needs of persons facing a bone marrow, blood, or umbilical cord stem cell blood transplant. A team of highly qualified medical experts reviews all medical information that appears on this Web site to insure accuracy.

If a stem cell, bone marrow, or cord blood transplant is in your future, BMTIN may be able to help. Since 1990, BMTIN is reported to have provided quality information and emotional support to more than 100,000 transplant patients, survivors and their loved ones.

BMTIN network of transplant survivors is available to help newly diagnosed patients and their loved ones cope with the stress of a life-threatening diagnosis, and the prospect of a transplant.

Information sites provided include:
- Books
- Drug database
- Help us survive
- Helpful services
- News bulletin
- News letter
- Resource directory
- Search–for additional information

10.15   Breast Cancer Action
http://www.bcaction.org

Breast Cancer Action (BCA) is a grassroots group of ordinary people who have educated themselves on the facts and the issues related to breast cancer. They are committed to empowering women and men to participate fully in decision about diagnoses and treatment and to the precautionary principle of public health–first do no harm. BCA works with other organizations to encourage the use of environmentally safe alternative to ways of doing business that we know–or have reason to believe–are harmful.

Information services include sites for:

- Browse/search out newsletters
- Frequently asked questions
- Read our latest newsletter
- Special feature
- What's new

A Search site is provided to obtain information on topics of interest.

10.16 Breast Cancer Decision Guide
http://www.bcdg.org

The Breast Cancer Decision Guide (BCDG) was developed by the Department of Defense's Breast Cancer Prevention, Education and Diagnosis Program in December 1998. It is designed for individuals diagnosed with breast cancer and their family members. Its purpose is to provide reliable information and encourage communication among patients, doctors/healthcare providers, and family members, so that informed medical and non-medical decisions can be reached.

Users are cautioned that this web site does not provide medical advice and that all medical decisions should be made by you and your doctor.

Sites are provided for information on:

- Chemotherapy
- Clinical trials

- Complementary therapies
- Coping
  - Organizations, services, and other resources
  - Spanish language resources
- Decision Guide
- Diagnosis and prognosis
- General information
- Glossary
- Guidelines for breast cancer screening
- Hormonal therapy
- Interactive consultations
- Military- specific issues
- Overall treatment
- Radiation therapy
- Surgery
- Symptom management
- Transplant/bone marrow

Decision Guide provides information on results obtained from mammography and other imaging procedures, biopsy, specialized tests, and surgery as well as survival or recurrence statistics.

Diagnosis and Prognosis provides general information on:
- Biopsy
- Breast cancer types
- Determining cancer spread
- Factors affecting outcome

- Imaging
- Staging

For information more specific to your case, begin the Decision Guide Consultation: Information to Understand a Specific Breast Cancer Diagnosis

General Information provides information on a variety of breast cancer topics and links to other relevant topics.

Guidelines for Breast Cancer Screening, among other relevant information, cites the American Cancer Society Recommendations for Early Breast Cancer Detection.

- Breast self-exam–monthly for all women 20 and over
- Clinical breast examination by a healthcare professional–every 3 years for women between ages 20-39 and every year for women aged 40 and over
- Screening mammography–every year for women aged 40 and over

Interactive Consultation provides information pertinent to your own diagnoses and personal situation. This is accomplished by asking for responses to questions on medical and non-medical factors that are important for making informed decisions. A biopsy or pathology report is regarded as helpful for answering some questions.

Treatment Decisions for Newly Diagnosed or Recurring Breast Cancer provides information on treatments that are considered appropriate, inappropriate, controversial and experimental. Information presented is derived from articles published in medical journals and oncology textbooks, and includes guidelines and the results of expert panels and surveys.

Connections to other sites are provided for additional information.

10.17   Breast Cancer Front Page
http://www.msnbc.com/news/BRCANCER_front.asp

Breast Cancer Front Page (BCFP) features the latest news on breast cancer provided by MSNBC.com News. Click on "health" and then on "breast cancer" for desired information. News on the latest developments in breast cancer is made available on such topics as:

- Breast self-examination

- Prevention

- Screening/testing

- Support groups

- Treatment

  - Chemotherapy

  - New agents

  - Radiation therapy

  - Other therapies

A Search site is provided to obtain additional information.

10.18   Cancer Care
http://www.cancercare.org

Cancer Care (CC) a non-profit organization established in 1944, provides free professional help to people with breast cancer through counseling, education, information and referral and direct financial assistance. This organization is reported to have helped over one million people nation-wide through its toll-free Counseling Line and Teleconference Programs, office-based services and via the Web. Services are available to people of all ages at any stage of the disease. Cancer Care's activities extend to family members, caregivers, and professionals providing key information and assistance.

Sites are provided for information on:
- Cancer care services
- Cancer types
- Counseling
- Education programs
- Financial needs
- Helping hand guide
- Managing your cancer
- Newsletters
- Referring
- Teleconferences
- What's new in cancer care

A Search site is provided for obtaining additional information.

10.19 Cancer Education Breast Cancer Home Page
http://www.cancereducation.com

Cancer Education (CE) improves cancer care through the dissemination of up-to-date educational information for healthcare professionals, cancer patients, and their family members. Click on "Patient and Family Center" for patient information.

Featured sites include:
- Oncology Week in Review
- Patient and Family Center

- Professional Center

Search for breast cancer information via the "Patient and Family Center" and obtain the following types of information:

- Chemotherapy side effects
- Clinical trials
- Diagnosis and prognosis
- Live webcasts
- Medclips–audio and video news
- Medical resources
  - Bookstore
  - Dictionary
  - Drug information
  - Find a physician/treatment center
- Prevention
- Research findings
- Risk factors
- Screening
- Social issues
- Supportive issues
- Treatment
- Types of breast cancer

A Search site is provided for additional information.

10.20   Cancer Help–EduCare
http://www.cancerhelp.com/ed

EduCare is a breast health education website for women and their families. Books published by EduCare have received acclaimed reviews in the Journal of the National Cancer Institute. Click on "EduCare" and then "Visit EduCare Homepage".

This organization provides hospitals with consulting services for establishing comprehensive breast centers. Trains nurses as breast health educators/coordinators and furnishes customized educational materials for patients. Products and training are reported to be recognized internationally for excellence in meeting the educational and support needs of women and their families.

Patient Resources information sites include:

- Breast cancer
- Breast discharge
- Breast lump
- Breast pain
- Glossary
- Male breast cancer
- Partner support
- Recurrent diagnosis
- Spiritual aspects

Clinical Resources information sites feature:
- Articles
- Breast centers

- Consulting
- RN training
- Slide presentations
- Teaching sheets

A Search site is provided to obtain additional information.

EduCare's "Recurrent Breast Cancer Report" is available free of charge. Patient Teaching Sheets on Breast Health and Breast Cancer also are made available.

10.21   Cancer News
http://www.cancernews.com

Cancer News (CN) provides the latest information on cancer prevention, diagnosis and treatment. Click on "breast cancer" for current news and information.

Information sites featured include:
- Books on breast cancer
- Breast cancer answers
- Breast cancer information center–general information, diagnosis, mammography, prevention, treatment, support groups and insurance issues
- Breast cancer literature search–link to National Library of Medicine's search engine and other related databases.
- Breast cancer network–latest news and articles plus links to other related sites and resources.
- Breast cancer section of MSNBC

- Breast cancer young women–effect of chemotherapy on ovarian function, fertility, and birth defects
- Clinical trials search
- Ladies first–post-mastectomy products including silicone breast forms
- National Breast Cancer Coalition
- National Cancer Institute–breast cancer risks, menopausal hormonal replacement therapy and tamoxifen
- Oncology drug reviews–link to the Medical Sciences Bulletin site which provides informative reviews on various cancer drugs
- Research update from Yahoo News
- Self-examination–Memorial Sloan Kettering Cancer Center site
- Sentinel node biopsy–to evaluate spread to lymph nodes
- Staging and treatment–links to NCI sites
- Stereotactic breast surgery
- Support groups
- Tamoxifen–questions and answers–link to NIH document
- Tamoxifen/raloxifene NCI study–comparative effects women at increased risk

A Search site is provided to obtain latest breast cancer news on topics of interest.

10.22 Cancer Research Foundation of America
http://www.crfa.org

The Cancer Research Foundation of America (CRFA), founded in 1985, is a national non-profit health foundation that focuses on cancers that can be prevented through lifestyle changes or early detection followed by prompt treatment. These include breast, cervical, colorectal, lung, prostate, skin and testicular cancers, which account for the majority of all cancer diagnoses and cancer-related deaths.

Click on "Women's Health" for details of how to conduct a breast self-exam in front of a mirror, lying down, and in the shower. This three-step exam may be done every month, 5-7 days after the beginning of your period. If you don't have a period, simply choose a specific day each month to do the exam. Report findings to your healthcare provider.

A search site is provided for information on breast cancer topics of interest by age groups.

Featured information sites include:
- Breast cancer decline rate validates screening research
- Breast cancer guide book supports breast cancer research
- Breast ductal lavage may help women better predict breast cancer
- Clinical trials
- Eating fruits and vegetables may protect against breast cancer
- Links to other breast cancer sites
- NCI announces first major trial of digital mammography
- Reports suggest an active lifestyle may protect against breast cancer
- Smoking increases breast cancer risks
- Support organizations
- Surgery and chemo prevention may lower the risk for women with BRCA mutations

10.23 Cancer Source
http://www.cancersource.com

Cancer Source (CS), founded in 1999, provides access to a full range of cancer resources. Their Medical Advisory board is led by Vincent De Vita, Director of the Yale Cancer Center, and other leading oncology professionals who ensure the reliability and timeliness and accuracy of the information provided.

Click on "cancer types" and then on "breast cancer" to arrive at "Breast Cancer Home". Here you will find a wealth of information and resources related specifically to breast cancer.

Click on "breast cancer news" to obtain latest developments.

Click on "learn more about breast cancer" and obtain information on:
- Care issues
- Disease overview - what is breast cancer, statistics, risk factors, prevention, screening, symptoms, pathophysiology, diagnosis, staging and classification
- Exercise
- Living with cancer
- Questions and answers
- Research
- Sexual relationships
- Symptom management, side effects
- Treatment options, types, goals, surgery, chemotherapy, radiotherapy, hormonal therapy

Click on "estimating breast cancer risk" to find a Breast Cancer Risk Assessment Tool–a computer program that women and their healthcare provider can use to estimate a woman's chance of developing breast cancer.

Features other information sites for

- Cancer glossary
- Cancer live chats
- Feature articles

A Search site is provided for additional information of interest.

10.24   Centers for Disease Control and Prevention
   http://www.cdc.gov

The Centers for Disease Control and Prevention (CDC) is the lead Federal Agency for protecting the health and safety of people–at home and abroad. CDC serves as the national focus for developing and applying disease prevention and control, environmental health, and health promotion and education activities designed to improve the health of the people of the United States.

The CDC National Breast and Cervical Cancer Early Detection Program (NBCCEDP)–(http://www.cdc.gov/cancer/nbccedp) established in 1991 provides:

- Breast and cervical cancer screening services to women who are low income and to racial/ethnic minorities and older women
- Linkages
- Monitoring of the quality of the screening process
- Public information and education programs to increase screening services

- Referrals, and when necessary, appropriate diagnostic follow-up, case management and assurances for medical treatment
- Services health professionals to improve the screening processes
- Surveillance and epidemiological controls

Approximately 2 million women have taken advantage of services provided through NBCCEDP but this constitutes only about 15% of the eligible population. Efforts are currently being made to step up the commitment to reach all eligible women.

A CDC Search site is provided for obtaining available information on topics of interest. For example, in searching "breast cancer", information is made available on:

- Diagnosis and treatment
- Environmental effects
- Facts/statistics
- Genetic influences
- Mammography benefits/recommendations
- Oral contraceptive use and risk
- Prevention
- Prophylactic bilateral mastectomy
- Risk factors

Use this search site to obtain additional information.

10.25 Centerwatch Clinical Trials Listing Service
http://www.centerwatch.com

Center Watch (CW) is a Boston-based publishing company that provides information services about clinical trials. It has an extensive list of

Institutional Review Board (IRB) approved clinical trials being conducted internationally.

Information is provided on a listing of more than 40,000 pharmaceutical industry and government-sponsored clinical trials. It is a site designed as a resource both for patients interested in participating in clinical trials and for research professionals.

Their Web site also lists promising new therapies recently approved by the Food and Drug Administration (FDA).

10.26   Clinical Trials.gov
http://www.clinicaltrials.gov

The U.S. National Institute of Health, through its National Library of Medicine has developed Clinical Trials.gov to provide patients, family members and members of the public current information about clinical research studies in breast cancer and other diseases.

This site was launched in February 2000 and currently lists approximately 5,700 clinical studies sponsored by the National Institute of Health, other Federal agencies, and the pharmaceutical industry in over 63,000 locations worldwide. Studies listed in the database are conducted primarily in the United States and Canada, but include locations in about 70 countries.

You may Search Clinical Trials, Search by Specific Information, Browse by Condition and/or Sponsor, and obtain further Resource Information via:

- Healthfinder–consumer health and human services information
- Medlineplus–authoritative consumer health information
- NIH Health Information–research sponsored by the National Institutes of Health

- Understanding Clinical Trials–information explaining and describing clinical trials

10.27 CNN.com/Health (Cable News Network)
http://www.cnn.com/Health

An AOL Time Warner Company cable news network. Breast Cancer information is provided by WebMD in conjunction with the prestigious Cleveland Clinic in Cleveland, Ohio.

For information, click on "breast cancer" under "community" and go to the "Breast Cancer Center" page to "Your Guide to Breast Cancer" by the Cleveland Clinic.

Featured information sites include:
- Breast Health
  - Anatomy of the breast
  - How to do a self-exam
  - Types of benign breast lumps
  - What to expect from your Doctor's exam
- Clinical Trials
- Detection
  - Bone densitometry scan
  - Breast biopsy
  - Mammogram
  - MRI
  - Sentinel node biopsy
  - Ultrasound
- Diet and fitness

- Know the Basics
  - Basics about breast cancer
  - Male breast cancer
- Mammography Saves Lives
- Newly diagnosed
- Risks and prevention
  - Genetics/testing
  - Hormone replacement therapy
  - Preventive breast cancer surgery
  - Risk factors
  - Screening guidelines
- Self-Exam
  - How to do a Breast Self-exam
  - What Should I Do if I Find a Lump
  - When Should I Perform a Breast Self-Exam
  - What to Expect from Your Doctor's Exam
- Treatment options
  - Bone marrow transplantation
  - Breast implants
  - Breast reconstruction surgery
  - Cancer-related fatigue
  - Chemotherapy
  - Radiation
- We Know You'd Want to Know
- Your follow-up care
  - Breast cancer during pregnancy

- Follow-up care
- How to cope
- Lymphedema
- Recurrence
- Self-exam after treatment

A Search site is provided to obtain additional information.

10.28 Coalition of National Cancer Cooperative Groups
http://www.cancertrialshelp.org

The Coalition of National Cancer Cooperative Groups (CNCCG) is a premier network of cancer clinical trials specialists. Members include cooperative groups, cancer centers, academic medical centers, community hospitals, physician practices, and patient advocate groups. Together they represent the interests of more than 12,000 cancer investigators, hundreds of patient advocates and thousands of patients worldwide.

Cancer clinical trials are regarded as one of the most important weapons in the continuing fight against cancer in order to improve the quality of life and the survival of people with cancer. CNCCG aims to insure the continued opportunity for cancer patients to participate in quality clinical trials.

Featured information sites include:
- Clinical trial ABC's
- Clinical trial list
- Health professionals
- Patient advocate
- Patient/family member/caregiver

Links to other related sites are available. A Search site is provided to obtain additional information of interest.

10.29   FDA Office of Women's Health
http://www.fda.gov/womens/default.htm

The Office of Women's Health (OWH) of the Food and Drug Administration was founded in 1994 to serve women's health objectives through program activities with government and non-government entities including consumer groups, health advocates, professional organizations, and industry.

Major Program Activities include:

- Funding research in pressing women's issues such as breast cancer.
- Education about safe medicine use in women
- Encouraging participation of women in breast cancer clinical trials
- Advocating for women's health and raising awareness and focus on breast cancer
- Providing information on breast cancer to Congress, the press, health professionals, women's health advocates, and the lay public in a variety of ways

The Health Topic site provides relevant information on:

- Breast cancer
  - Better treatments save more lives
  - Cancer liaison program of the FDA Office of Special Health Issues
  - Tamoxifen
- Breast implants
  - Choosing a surgeon

- Frequently asked questions
- Guidelines
- Immunologic effects of silicone breast implants
- Issues to consider/risks
- Status report on breast implant safety
- Surgical aspects
- Reconstruction with implants
- Reconstruction with implants: tissue flap procedure
- Mammography
  - FDA's mammography program
  - FDA sets higher standards for mammography

The Search site allows the user to obtain additional information.

10.30   Guide to Quality Breast Cancer Care
http://www.natlbcc.org/nbccf/info/main.html

Obtaining and using the right information can significantly affect your health and healthcare. To be well informed about breast cancer and make wise health care choices, the Guide to Quality Breast Cancer Care (GQBCC) developed by the National Breast Cancer Coalition (NBCC) is regarded as useful. Click on "Patient Guide" to obtain a copy.

Further information sites include:
- Complimentary and alternative medicine
- Current evidence-based breast guidelines
- Diagnosis and treatment
- Medical research/clinical trials
- "Natural" does not always mean "safe"

- Risk factors/prevention
- Second opinion
- Standard care
- Surgery and radiation
- Take charge, control, responsibility for your health and healthcare
- Things you should know when evaluating medical information/resources on the Web

10.31   Harvard Medical School
http://www.hms.harvard.edu

The Harvard Medical School (HMS) site provides quality information by Intelihealth. Medical content of this site is reviewed by the faculty of the Harvard Medical School to assure that the information provided is current, comprehensive, and useful.

Harvard Medical School is one of the world's preeminent institutions in medical education, patient care, and research. The breadth and depth of its scientific and clinical disciplines are unsurpassed. The school has nearly 8000 faculty and 17 affiliated facilities.

Click on "InteliHealth" featuring the Harvard Medical Schools community health information.

Click on "Diseases and Conditions" and then on "Breast Cancer". Information sites featured include:
- What is it
  - Description
  - Diagnosis
  - Main forms

- Prevention
- Prognosis
- Symptoms
- Statistics
- Risk factors
  - Alcohol
  - Environmental factors
  - Estrogen connection
  - Family history
  - Genetics
  - Shift work
  - Smoking
  - Stronger bones, more breast cancer
  - Weight
- Diagnosis and screening
  - Early detection is the key
  - Importance of breast self-exam
  - Role of mammograms
  - Size of cancer is crucial
  - Types of breast cancer and their prognosis
  - Types of breast cancer biopsy (core, stereotactic, surgical)
- Staging and treatment
  - Chemotherapy
  - Hormonal therapy
  - Lumpectomy
  - Lymph nodes

- Mastectomy
- Radiation
- Staging
- Tamoxifen
- Expert commentary
  - Hormone therapy
  - The pill
- News/research reviews

  December 2001

  § Bilateral mastectomy for BRCA-1 and BRCA-2 mutations

  § Breast cancer risk with hormone use

  § Intake of soy food compounds and risk

  § Lifetime activity and risk

  § Weight as a factor

  November 2001

  § Chemotherapy survival

  § Conservative surgery for ductal carcinoma in situ

  § Folate use and risk

  § Survival in hereditary breast cancer

  § Thyroid cancer increases risk

  October 2001

  § Breast feeding and reduced risk

  § Chemotherapy and bone loss

  § Fruits and vegetables and risk

  September 2001

  § Hormone replacement therapy and recurrence

§ Letrozole more effective than tamoxifen for advanced disease

<u>August 2001</u>

§ Breast implants and risk, detection, and survival

§ Environmental pollutants and risks

§ Pain killers and breast cancer

§ Soy and breast cancer risk

<u>July 2001</u>

§ Alcohol and risk

§ Inactivity, weight gain and chemotherapy

§ Low risk of recurrence patients benefit from adjuvant treatment

<u>June 2001</u>

§ Determining breast cancer without surgery

§ Recurrence in ductal carcinoma in situ

§ Tamoxifen lack of effect on psychological and sexual well being

§ Tamoxifen treatment beyond five years

<u>May 2001</u>

§ Benefit of breast cancer centers on disease management

§ Breast conserving therapy

§ Lower bone mineral density and risk

§ Risk of breast cancer lower than women think

§ Risk of colorectal cancer not increased in breast cancer survivors

<u>April 2001</u>

§ Breast reduction surgery and risk

§ Health problems in older women with breast cancer

§ Personality factors and risk

March 2001

§ Breast fed and risk

§ Surgery choices in older women

§ Reconstruction option

§ Fruits and vegetables and risk

§ Exercise benefits

February 2001

§ Breast density increases with HRT reversible

§ Drug fails to prevent breast cancer from spreading

§ Chemotherapy regimen for metastatic breast cancer

§ Women with small breasts and chemotherapy

January 2001

§ Acupuncture and nausea and vomiting

§ Breast cancer in women with a history of cancer

§ Patients view of lymph node surgery

Use the sites "Harvard Medical Web" or the Search site for additional information of interest.

10.32   Health On the Net Foundation
http://www.hon.ch

The Health On the Net Foundation (HON), created in 1995, is a not-for-profit international organization located in Geneva, Switzerland that provides current, comprehensive, and useful international health information. The major sponsors of HON are the Swiss Institute of Bioinformatics, the State of Geneva, Switzerland, and the Geneva University Hospital.

HON also provides leadership in establishing ethical standards for Web site providers. The HON Code of Conduct and eight ethical management principles for healthcare Web sites is available in 19 languages.

Free and unlimited access to Medline from the National Library of Medicine, USA databases is made available for in depth Search purposes.

HON also provides its own Search site for world wide search for "breast cancer" information from its own database. Information is provided by site source and location, degree of relevance to topic searched, language, and date.

10.33   Healthfinder
http://www.healthfinder.gov

Healthfinder is the U.S. Department of Health and Human Services Website for current, comprehensive, and useful information. It features a Health Library of handpicked information A to Z on prevention, wellness, diseases and conditions, and alternative/complementary medicine plus a medical dictionary, encyclopedia, journals and more. Their Directory of Healthfinder Organizations features carefully selected Web Resources from government agencies, clearinghouses, nonprofit foundations and universities.

Click on "Diseases and Conditions" and go to "Breast cancer". This site provides information/reports on a variety of subjects such as:

- Abortion and breast cancer–increased risk after an induced abortion

- Adjuvant therapy–more treatment options a better chance for long-term survival for invasive cancer

- Breast cancer–overview provided by Net Wellness and a glossary of breast cancer terms

- Breast cancer decision guide–interactive consultation page provided by the Office of the Secretary of Defense
- *Breast Cancer: Better Treatments Save More Lives*–an article on options available from Consumer Information Center, U.S. General Services Administration
- Male breast cancer–general overview by Y-Me National Breast Cancer Organization
- National Action Plan on Breast Cancer–provided by the U.S. Public Health Service's Office on Women's Health
- Screening–from the NCI
- Facts about mammograms–from the NCI
- Comprehensive listing of resources and information for the consumer, patient and health care provider offered in both Spanish and English by NOAH: New York Online Access of Health
- Breast cancer and the environment–risk factors and environmental agents from the National Institute of Environmental Health Sciences
- Improving methods of detection and diagnosis–*Mammography and Beyond* published by the National Academy Press
- Male breast cancer — treatment information for healthcare professionals from the National Cancer Institutee
- Menopause - treatment options for women concerned about estrogen replacement therapy summary report by experts from the Hormone Foundation
- National Cancer Institute–overview, screening, prevention, risk factors, treatment options, clinical trials, genetics and more
- What you need to know about breast cancer–screening and early detection, symptoms, diagnosis, treatment and rehabilitation and more from the National Cancer Institute
- Questions to ask your doctor about mammography–from the NCI

- Reach to Recovery Program–visitation program by trained volunteers providing information and support to women with breast cancer by American Cancer Society

- Study of Tamoxifen versus Raloxifene (STAR) - breast cancer prevention study

- Preventive mastectomy–removal of one or both breasts to prevent or reduce risk of breast cancer in genetically susceptible women from the NCI

- Ask NOAH About: Breast Cancer–comprehensive consumer health information about breast cancer by NOAH: New York Online Access to Health

- FAQ: About Tamoxifen–answers to concerns most women have about tamoxifen from the NCI

- Mammograms: Not Just Once, But For a Lifetime–basic consumer information concerning the benefits of mammography screening from the NCI

- Self-care flow charts - breast problems in women

- Understanding Breast Changes: A Health Guide For All Women - provides a description of screening methods for the early detection of breast cancer and the various types of breast changes that women experience throughout life.

- Your Cancer Risk–assessment tool for estimating and lowering their risk of the 12 most common cancers from the Education Institute

A Search site is provided for additional information.

10.34 Imaginis Breast Health Specialists
http://www.imaginis.com

Imaginis Breast Health Specialists is an information resource for patients and health care professionals on breast health and breast cancer. Imaginis provides women and their physicians with relevant information created by an independent team of experts to insure that it is up-to-date and accurate.

Breast cancer information sites featured include:

- Breast Biopsy
- Clinical trials
- Diagnosis
- Drugs
- Glossary
- Hormone therapy
- Imaging
- Medical procedures
- Myths
- Online medical journals
- Pain
- Practice Guidelines
- Professional discussion, resources
- Reconstructive surgery
- Resources and support
- Self-exam
- Teaching files

A Search site is provided to obtain further information.

10.35 Johns Hopkins Breast Center
http://www.med.jhu.edu/breastcenter

The Johns Hopkins Breast Center, of the Johns Hopkins Hospital and Johns Hopkins Medical School, is at the forefront of breast cancer research and treatment. The Center's state-of-the-art technology and highly skilled medical professionals are internationally recognized. The Breast Center has a comprehensive, multi-disciplinary breast cancer program, offering a full spectrum of clinical and support services, from screening and diagnosis to treatment and counseling.

Information sites are provided for:
- Artemis- latest information on research and other issues of importance
- Contact a professional, speak with a survivor, or obtain information about services
- Educational information
- Guides to Breast Cancer Diagnosis and Treatment
- Nutrition
- Pathology
- Patient care
- Research highlights
- Resources for patient/professionals
- Support programs
  - Chatroom
  - Listen to our survivors
  - Patient/ family support
  - Related links
- Testimonials

- Treatment and diagnosis
  - Making the right decisions for you
  - Patient bill of rights
  - Post-treatment issues
  - Survivor retreats

10.36   Komen Breast Center Foundation
http://www.komen.org

The Komen Foundation features Breast Cancerinfo.com, a comprehensive, reliable source for information. This site provides fact sheets as well as a powerful search engine that provides users with in-depth scientific information about a variety of topics. BreastCancerinfo.com also includes a comprehensive registry of community organizations, programs and educational materials with contact information and/or links to connect users with resources they need.

Information sites are featured for:

- Komen Facts for Life–basic facts from early detection to support, a glossary of questions and answers, facts and statistics
- The Komen site "About Breast Cancer: The ABCs of Breast Cancer" - co-developed with the Harvard Center for Cancer Prevention. It is reported to provide current reliable information on:
  - Introduction–an overview
  - Breast Cancer–a review
  - What Increases the Chance–risk factors
  - Early Detection–issues related to screening and early detection
  - Diagnosis–current standard of practice in diagnoses and descriptions of prognostic and predictive factors

- Staging–TNM method of staging
- Treating–current standard of practice in treating early stage, locally advanced, and metastatic breast cancer.
- Complementary Cancer Therapies–types of complementary therapies available to patients
- Getting Good Care–a review of the components that makeup quality medical care
- After Treatment–Living with Cancer–follow-up care and behaviors that may improve outcome
- Social support–strategies for finding support groups, helping families cope
- Financing–financing medical care
- Resources–organizations and information sources that can provide additional information.
- Glossary–definitions of terminology used

A Search site is provided to obtain additional information.

10.37 Mautner Project
http://www.mautnerproject.org

Founded in 1990, the Mautner Project is a national organization dedicated to lesbians with cancer, their partners and caregivers. This organization offers:

- Direct services to lesbians, their partners and caregivers
- Education information to the lesbian community
- Education to the health care community about the special concerns of lesbians and their families
- Advocacy on lesbian health issues in national and local arenas

Features breast cancer information sites on:

- What's new
- Program
- Support services
    - Family services
    - Support groups
    - Phone support
- Resources
    - Resource center
    - Outreach and education
    - Advocacy
- Statistics on breast cancer
- What puts women at risk
    - Smoking
    - Family history
    - Reproductive history
    - Diet
    - Socioeconomic
    - Factors
    - Age
- Be aware of warning signs of breast cancer
- Monthly breast self-exam
    - In the shower
    - Before a mirror
    - Lying down

- In a circle
- Standing
- Disclaimer
- Sister sites/links
- Spanish language information site is available

10.38 Mayo Clinic and Foundation
http://www.mayo.edu

Mayo Clinic and Foundation is a not-for-profit organization located in Rochester, Minnesota, with branches in Arizona and Florida. More than 2,000 physicians and 35,000 allied health staff work in the Mayo system, treating nearly a half million patients annually. Comprehensive, reliable information is made available through their database and key links to other sources.

Click on "Health and Medical Information" and then on "Diseases and Conditions A-Z" and then on "Breast Cancer" for desired information. Sites featured are:
- Additional resources
- Biological therapy
- Biopsy
- Breast calcium deposits
- Breast cancer in men
- Breast self-examination
- Cancer center
- Causes
- Chemotherapy
- Clinical trials
- Coping
- Genetic testing

- Hormone therapy
- Intimacy
- Lumpectomy
- Mammograms
- Modified radical mastectomy
- Oral contraceptives
- Partial/segmental mastectomy
- Prevention
- Radiation therapy
- Receptor tests—estrogen and progesterone
- Reconstructive surgery
- Reconstruction of your nipple and areola
- Reconstruction with implants
- Reconstruction with your own tissue
- Risk factors
- Screening and diagnosis
- Sentinel lymph node biopsy
- Signs and symptoms
- Staging
- Strong support system
- Surgery/Simple mastectomy
- Taking care of yourself
- Taking control
- Telling others
- Treatment
- Ultrasound
- What is breast cancer
- When to seek medical advice

Information also is made available in the Spanish language.

A Search site is provided for obtaining additional information.

10.39 Medlineplus
http://www.medlineplus.gov

A service of the National Library of Medicine, National Institutes of Health. Features sites on:

- Health topics–conditions, diseases and a medical encyclopedia
- Drugs–generic and brand name
- Dictionaries–spellings and definitions of medical terms
- Directories–doctors and hospitals
- Other resources–organizations, consumer health libraries, international sites, publications, Medline and more

Click on "Health Topics" and then on "B" for breast cancer information sites including:

- Clinical trials
- Coping
- Diagnosis/symptoms
- Dictionaries/glossaries
- General/overview
- Male breast cancer
- National Institutes of Health
- News articles
- Organizations
- Pictures/diagrams
- Prevention/screening
- Research findings
- Spanish language information
- Specific conditions/aspects

- Statistics
- Treatment

A Spanish language information site is available

A Search site is made available for additional information.

10.40   National Academy Press
http://www.nap.edu

Mammography and Beyond: Developing Technologies for the Early Detection of Breast Cancer by Sheryl J. Nass, I. Craig Henderson, and Joyce C. Lashof, editors; National Cancer Policy Board, Institute of Medicine and Commission on Life Sciences, National Research Council published by the National Academy Press, 2101 Constitution Avenue, N.W., Box 285, Washington, DC 20055, 2001, pp 288. The full text of this report is available on line from the National Academy Press at: http:www.nap.edu.

Search for "Mammography and Beyond" and read it free on line. The Open Book page is a browsable, nonproprietary, fully and deeply searchable version of the publication.

Contents of the book include:
- Executive summary
- Breast imaging and related technologies
- Technologies in development: genetics and tumor markers
- Development and regulation of new technologies
- Evaluation and cost coverage of new technologies
- Dissemination: increasing use and availability of new technologies
- Findings and recommendations

10.41   National Alliance of Breast Cancer Organizations
http://www.nabco.org

The National Alliance of Breast Cancer Organizations (NABCO) is a non-profit information and education resource on breast cancer comprised of a network of over 400 member organizations nationwide. NABCO provides information to medical professionals and their organizations and to patients and their families, and advocates.

Features sites on:

- Advanced breast cancer

- Books

- Clinical trials

- Latest information: NABCO News

- Research

- Resource list

- Support groups in your area

NABCO Resource List 2001/02 is a listing of over 3,000 resources for the breast cancer community consisting of books, brochures, booklets, organizations, websites and local support groups. These resources cover such topics as general information about breast cancer, making treatment choices, support for patients and family members, and planning for end of life. Over 850 support groups located in every state, the District of Columbia and Canada are included.

10.42   National Breast Cancer Coalition
http://www.natlbcc.org

The National Breast Cancer Coalition (NBCC) founded in 1991, consists of a network of activists across the USA consisting of more than 500 organizations and 60,000 individuals strong.

Provides useful breast cancer report entitled "Guide to Quality Breast Cancer Care".

10.43   National Cancer Institute
http://www.nci.nih.gov
http://www.cancer.gov

The National Cancer Institute (NCI) of the National Institutes of Health (NIH) is the premier U.S. government effort and resource regarding cancer. It provides current, comprehensive and useful cancer information for both patients and healthcare professionals. In January 2002, the NCI launched an improved, easy-to-use one-stop resource for cancer information at: http://www.cancer.gov.

Go to this one-stop resource for desired information, click on "types of cancer" and subsequently on "breast cancer" which will take you to the "Breast Cancer Home Page". This site provides you with information on a variety of breast cancer topics including:

- What You Need to Know About Breast Cancer
- PDQ (Physicians' Data Query) Reports–NCI's comprehensive cancer database

Information is made available in the English and Spanish languages.

"What You Need to Know About Breast Cancer" provides information regarding the following topics:

- Biopsy
- Breast cancer: who's at risk
- Breast reconstruction
- Causes and prevention
- Chemotherapy
- Detection and diagnosis
- Detecting breast cancer
- Diagnosing breast cancer
- Follow-up care
- Hormonal therapy
- Introduction
- Methods of treating breast cancer
- National Cancer Institute booklets
- National Cancer Institute Information Resources
- Planning treatment
- Radiation therapy
- Recognizing symptoms
- Rehabilitation
- Second opinion
- Side effects of treatment
- Support for women with breast cancer
- Surgery
- The breasts
- The promise of cancer research

- Treatment
- Treatment choices
- Understanding the cancer process
- When cancer is found

PDQ provides peer-reviewed summaries on breast cancer treatment, screening, prevention, genetics and support care, among other topics. A registry of over 12,000 cancer clinical trials from around the world, directories of physicians and professionals and genetic services, and organizations that provide cancer care/information also are provided. Current literature from more than 70 biomedical journals are reviewed for relevant information and this is synthesized into clear summaries for reports.

Separate sites are provided for:
- Female breast cancer
- Breast cancer and pregnancy
- Male breast cancer

Breast Cancer: Who's at Risk site provides information on:
- Abortion and breast cancer - no relationship
- Antiperspirants/deodorants–no relationship
- Diagnostic x-rays–x-rays prior to 1970 for scoliosis increases breast cancer mortality
- Diethystilbesterol use by mother–no relationship
- Environmental tobacco smoke–see report for findings
- Estrogen and progesterone–greater risk of breast cancer with combination compared to estrogen alone
- Heterocyclic amines in cooked meats–see report for findings

- Magnetic field exposures - no apparent effect
- Menopausal hormone replacement therapy—see report for findings
- Oral contraceptives—see report for findings
- Silicone breast implants—not linked to breast cancer risk

Detecting/Screening site offers information on:
- Breast cancer screening/detection
- Breast cancer and mammography
- FDA approval of breast imaging devices
- FDA certified mammography facilities
- Improved imaging methods for breast cancer detection and diagnosis
- Interpreting laboratory test trials
- NCI's sentinel node biopsy trials
- Screening mammograms: questions and answers
- Tumor markers
- Understanding breast changes: a health guide for all women

Treatment sites provide information on a variety of topics including:
- Adjuvant therapy
- Biological therapies
- Bone marrow transplantation, peripheral blood stem cell transplantation
- Chemotherapy
- Early breast cancer
- Herceptin (trastuzumab)
- High dose chemotherapy
- Inflammatory breast cancer

- Metastatic breast cancer
- Radiation plus tamoxifen
- Radiation therapy
- Screening and testing
- Sentinel node biopsy trials
- Shortened radiation schedule
- Surgical therapy
- Taxanes
- Tamoxifen
- Understanding breast cancer treatment: a guide for patients

Clinical Trials site contains information on:
- Breast cancer updates (news)
- PDQs database
- Search NCI's clinical trails database
- STAR trial (tamoxifen vs. raloxifene)

CancerLit is a bibliographic database that contains more than 1.5 million citations and abstracts from over 4,000 different sources including bio-medical journals, proceedings, books, reports, and doctoral theses. The database contains references to cancer literature published from the 1960s to the present and is updated with more than 8,000 records every month.

Topic searches includes information on:
- Chemotherapy
- Radiotherapy
- Screening and prevention
- Surgery for breast cancer

CancerLit site provides sites for:

- Breast cancer genetics
- Cancerlit database
- Cancerlit Breast Cancer Topic searches
  - Diagnosis
  - Prevention
  - Treatment
- Chromosome 13 in hereditary breast cancer
- Directory of breast cancer genetics professionals who provide services related to genetic risk assessment, counseling and testing
- Hereditary and non-hereditary breast cancers
- Overview

Related Information site contains reports on:

- Breast Cancer Progress Review Group
- Metastatic Breast Cancer: Questions and Answers

Support and Resources site has relevant information on:

- Finances
- Hospice
- Home care
- Support organizations

Statistics site provides information on:

- Probability of breast cancer in American women
- Statistical data sources
- U.S. racial/ethnic cancer patterns

Coping with Cancer site has information on side effects and complications of beast cancer and its treatment for patients, survivors and caregivers. Emotional Concerns contains information on:

- Anxiety
- Depression
- Loss, grief and bereavement
- Post traumatic stress disorder
- Sexuality
- Substance abuse

Understanding Clinical Trials site has reports on:

- Benefits from taking part
- How they work
- Risks
- Types of trials

Complementary and Alternative Medicine site provides information regarding:

- Healing philosophies
- Approaches and therapies used in addition to, or instead of, traditional treatments

A Search site also is provided for obtaining additional information.

10.44 National Center for Complementary and Alternative Medicine
http://www.nccam.nih.gov

The National Center for Complementary and Alternative Medicine (NCCAM) at the National Institutes of Health (NIH) evaluates complementary and alternative medicine (CAM) healing practices and disseminates authoritative information.

CAM covers a broad range of healing philosophies (schools of thought), approaches, and therapies that mainstream Western (conventional) medicine does not commonly use, accept, study, understand, or make available. CAM practices may include such things as the use of acupuncture, herbs, homeopathy, therapeutic massage and traditional oriental medicine to promote well being or treat health conditions

CAM treatments may be used alone, as an alternative to conventional therapies, or in addition to conventional, mainstream therapies, in what is referred to as a complementary or an integrative approach. CAM therapies are sometimes called holistic, meaning that they consider the whole person including physical, mental, emotional, and spiritual aspects.

A status report on clinical trials of phytoestrogens and breast cancer is provided

The user is cautioned not to use the CAM therapies described on these Web pages without consulting a licensed healthcare provider.

A Search site is provided to obtain information on complementary and alternative medicine as it may pertain to breast cancer.

10.45 National Coalition for Cancer Survivorship
http://www.cansearch.org

The National Coalition for Cancer Survivorship (NCCS) was founded in 1986 as a patient led advocacy organization working on behalf of people with all types of cancer and their families. NCCS works for quality cancer care for all Americans by leading and strengthening the survivorship movement, empowering cancer survivors, and advocating for policy issues that affect cancer survivors' quality of life.

Sites are featured for information on:
- Cancer: keys to survivorship
  - Communication and fighting fatigue
  - Living with, through and beyond cancer
  - Strategies for self-care
  - What are keys to survivorship
  - What cancer survivors need to know about health insurance
  - Working it out: employment rights
- Cancer survival toolbox
- Cansearch websites
- Conferences and events
- Minority cancer survivorship programs
- NCCS town halls
- Public health policy issues
- Search site for additional information
- Spirituality committee
- Survivorship programs
- What's new

10.46   National Hospice Foundation
http://www.hospiceinfo.org

The National Hospice Foundation (NAF), a charitable organization, was created in 1992 to broaden American's understanding of hospice through research and education. Its mission is to expand America's vision for end-of-life care.

NHF engages and informs the public about a quality end-of-life care that hospice provides.

Features information sites for:
- What is hospice and how to select a hospice program
  - What is hospice care
  - How does hospice care work
  - How do I go about choosing a hospice
  - What kind of services should I expect from a hospice
  - How does hospice care begin
  - What kind of support is available to the family/caregiver
  - What role does the physician play
  - Will I be the only hospice patient that the hospital staff serve
  - What role does the hospice volunteer serve
  - What does the hospice do to keep the patient comfortable
  - Is hospice available after hours
  - Can I be cared for by hospice if I reside in a nursing home, etc
  - What happens if I cannot stay at home
  - How do I insure that quality care is provided
  - Do State and Federal reviewers inspect and evaluate hospices

- Do I pay for hospice care
- When is the right time to ask about hospice
- Question checklist
- Consumer brochures
  - Hospice Care: A Consumer's Guide to Selecting a Hospice Program
  - Communicating Your End-of-Life Wishes
  - Hospice Care and the Medicare Hospice Benefit

10.47 National Library of Medicine
http://www.nlm.nih.gov

The National Library of Medicine (NLM) is the world's largest medical library and creator of other public and professional Web Resources such as Medline, PubMed, and Medlineplus.

Provides current, comprehensive, and useful information on:
- Clinicaltrials.gov–information for patients/professionals regarding clinical research studies/participation in
- General information–frequently asked questions and answers
- Medline, PubMed, and Medlineplus–breast cancer information selected for patients and professionals by NLM
- Library services–catalogues, databases, publications
- News
- Search site–to be used to obtain further information on:
  - Breast cancer
  - Breast diseases
  - Dictionaries/glossaries
  - Directories

- Doctors
- Drugs
- Hospitals
- Libraries
- Mammography
- Medical encyclopedia
- Medline
- Medlineplus
- Organizations
- Other resources

Information may be obtained in English, Spanish, or other languages on topics of interest. For example, if one searches "mammography", sites are made available for information on:

- Medline, Medlineplus and PubMed–recent articles, related pages on breast cancer, breast diseases, procedures and therapies
- Latest news–from United Press
- Screening mammograms from National Cancer Institute
- General/overviews on mammograms National Women's Health Information Center
- Mammography from American College of Radiology
- Pictures/diagrams–Atlas of the Body: The Breast–Disorders from the American Medical Association
- Research–best way to screen for breast cancer under debate from the National Cancer Institute
  - First major trial of digital mammography launched from the National Institutes of Health

- Study looks at reasons for false-positive mammograms from American Cancer Society
- Specific conditions/aspects–FDA approves first digital mammography system from Food and Drug Administration
- Dictionaries/glossaries
- Glossary from National Cancer Institute
- Directories–FDA Certified mammography facilities from the Center for Devices and Radiological Health, Food and Drug Administration
- Organizations–American Cancer Society and National Cancer Institute
- Statistics–mammography from National Center for Health Statistics

10.48 National Lymphedema Network
http://www.lymphnet.org

The National Lymphedema Network (NLN) is a non-profit organization founded in 1988 that provides education and guidance to patients, health care professionals and the general public by disseminating information on the prevention and management of primary and secondary lymphedema.

Provides sites for information on:
- Choosing a therapist
- Educational materials
- Guidelines
- Links
- Lymphlink
- Netpals and penpals
- Prevention
- Question corner/questionnaire

- Research
- Resource guide
- Support groups
- Volunteer

A Search site is provided for additional information of interest.

10.49 National Self-Help Clearinghouse
http://www.selfhelpweb.org

National Self-Help Clearinghouse (NSHC) a non profit organization founded in 1976, facilitates access to self-help groups and increases the awareness of the importance of mutual support.

The clearinghouse provides a number of services such as

- Assists human service agencies to integrate self-help principles
- Conducts training activities for self-help group leaders and professional facilitators of support groups
- Provides consultation to public agencies
- Carries out research about the effectiveness of self-help
- Provides information on self-help support groups and regional self-help clearinghouses
- Information on self-help and how does it work
- Search engines/links for self-help groups and local clearinghouses such as the "American Self-Help Clearinghouse"

The American Self-Help Clearinghouse (ASHC) puts people in touch with any of several hundred national and international self-help groups covering a wide range of illnesses such as "breast cancer". It has compiled a national database of over 800 of these and model groups. Referrals are provided to local self-help groups. ASHC also publishes the Self-Help Sourcebook, a listing of national group headquarters and model self-help groups, information on starting groups, and the availability of online computer support groups.

10.50   National Women's Health Information Center
http://www.4woman.gov

The National Women's Health Information Center (NWHIC) is the Office on Women's Health (OWH) clearinghouse for women's health information in the U.S. Department of Health and Human Service (DHHS). This site can help you download a wide variety of women's health related material developed by the Department of Health and Human Services under Federal agencies and private sector resources. They provide current, reliable health information to patients and their families.

The National Action Plan on Breast Cancer (http://www.4woman.gov/napbc) was designed to speed progress toward eradicating breast cancer.

A Search site is provided to obtain information of interest including:

- Clinical trials
- Frequently asked questions and answers
- Information in Spanish
- Information on the Web
- Organization and working groups
- Web stats
- What's New

10.51 NOAH: New York Online Access to Health
http://www.noah-health.org

NOAH is the combined effort of four key New York professional entities: the City University of New York, the Metropolitan New York Library Council, the New York Academy of Medicine and the New York Public Library. It serves the World Wide Web, provides information in English and Spanish, and is the recipient of numerous awards of excellence.

To obtain breast cancer information, first click on "Health Topics", then on "Cancer", and finally on "Breast Cancer" to arrive at the site entitled: "Ask NOAH: Breast Cancer".

NOAH utilizes breast cancer information from a variety of other key resources.

Sites are provided for information on the following breast cancer topics, among others:
- Basics
  - Facts
  - Guidelines
  - Glossary
  - Myths
  - Patients guidelines
  - Questions and answers
  - Types of breast cancer
  - Classification of breast cancer
  - Invasive breast cancer
  - Non-invasive breast cancer

- Paget's disease
- Staging and grading
- Care and treatment
  - Adjuvant therapy
  - Follow-up care
  - Guidelines
  - What's new
- Chemotherapy
  - Administration
  - Chemo prevention
  - Drugs used
  - High dose chemo
  - Mechanism of action
  - Questions and answers
  - Side effects
- Clinical trials
  - Things to know
  - Trial resources
- Diagnosis and prevention
  - Biopsy procedures
  - Clinical exam
  - Ductal lavage
  - Drugs to lower risk
  - Early detection
  - Lump evaluation
  - Mammography

- Outcome
- Prevention measures
- Questions and answers
- Self-exam
- Screening guidelines
- Ultrasound
- Diet and Prevention
  - Cancer prevention
  - Cancer and nutrition
- Information resources
- Risk factors and prevention
  - Abortion
  - Estrogen and progesterone
  - Genetics
  - Hormone replacement therapy
  - Oral contraceptives
  - Risk factors update
  - Tamoxifen and raloxifene
- Statistics
- Surgery
  - Breast conservation
  - Breast reconstruction
  - Choices
  - Lumpectomy
  - Lymph node dissection
  - Mastectomy

- Radiotherapy
  - Schedule of administration
  - Shortened radiation schedule
  - Side effects/coping
- Male breast cancer
  - Basics/What is it
  - Detection and symptoms
  - Overview and treatment
  - Prevention and risk factors
  - Statistics

10.52 Oncolink: University of Pennsylvania Cancer Center
http://www.oncolink.org

Oncolink was founded in 1994 by the University of Pennsylvania Cancer Center specialists to help cancer patients, families, health care professionals and the general public obtain accurate cancer related information at no charge. Comprehensive information is made available about specific types of cancer, updates on treatments, and news about research advances. Information is reported to be updated everyday and is provided at various levels, from introductory to in depth. For information on breast cancer, click on "Types of Cancer" and then on "Breast Cancer".

Sites are featured for information on:
- Description
  - What is beast cancer
  - Stages of breast cancer
  - Inflammatory breast cancer
  - Recurrent breast cancer

- Histological classification of breast cancer
- Treatment option overview
  - How breast cancer is treated
    - Surgery
    - Lumpectomy
    - Partial or segmental mastectomy
    - Other types of surgery
    - Radiation therapy
    - Radical mastectomy
    - Biological therapy
    - Bone marrow transplantation
    - Stem cell transplant
    - Treatment by stage
  - Ductal carcinoma in situ
  - Stage I, II and IIIa breast cancer
  - Stage IIIb and IV, recurrent, and metastatic breast cancer
- National Breast and Cervical Cancer Early Detection Program
- Overview of screening
  - What is screening
  - Breast cancer overview
  - Screening tests for breast cancer
  - Magnetic resonance imaging (MRI)
- Ask the experts answers to questions
  - Coping with cancer
  - Treatment options
  - Types of cancer

- Resources
- Implications of genetic breast cancer testing
- NCI Cancerlit
- NCI PDQ
- Coping with breast cancer
  - Caregivers
  - Hospice care
  - Nutrition during treatment
  - Sexuality
  - Side effects
  - Support
  - Survivorship
- Clinical trials
- Cancer resources
- Breast self examination
- Mammography
- Herceptin

10.53 Oncology Nursing Society
http://www.ons.org

Oncology Nursing Online (ONS), incorporated in 1975, is an information service for oncology nurses, other healthcare providers, people with cancer, and their families and friends. It is a national organization of more than 30,000 registered nurses and other healthcare professionals dedicated to excellence in patient care, teaching, research and education in the filed of oncology.

Features information sites on

- Evidence-based practice
- Research findings and resources
- Publications
- Online journals
- Bookstore
- Literature review
- News
- Cancer treatment news
- News from ONS journals
- The ONS News
- Clinical practice–a wealth of information about cancer prevention/detection, treatment, symptom management, survivorship and palliative care
- Education
- Cancerfatigue.org
- Cancer survival toolbox
- ONS resource center

10.54   Patient Advocate Foundation
http://www.patientadvocate.org

Patient Advocate Foundation (PAF) is a national non-profit organization that serves as an active liaison between that patient and insurer, employer and/or creditors to resolve insurance, job discrimination and/or debt crises matters relative to her diagnosis through managers, doctors and attorneys. PAF seeks to safeguard patients through effective mediation assuring access to healthcare, maintenance of employment and preservation of their financial stability.

Provides information sites on:

- Current issues
- Cancer news
- Clinical trials
- Patient resources
  - Mental health resources: guide for patient referrals
  - National legal resources network
  - National managed care network
  - Guidebook for patients: state by state directory
  - Your guide to the appeals process
  - Managed care answer guide
  - Patients in need of insurance, job discrimination, and debt crisis assistance
- Legal news
- Debt crisis intervention
- Job discrimination assistance
- Insurance issues and support
- Patient's bill of rights

A Search site is provided to obtain additional information.

10.55 Plastic Surgery Information Service
http://www.plasticsurgery.org

Plastic Surgery Information Service (PLIS) is sponsored by the American Society of Plastic Surgeons (ASPS) and the Plastic Surgery Educational

Foundation (PSEF). PLIS provides information on a variety of cosmetic and reconstructive plastic surgery procedures as well as offering a Plastic Surgeon Referral Service.

Sites are provided for:
- Find a plastic surgeon
- Surgical procedures
- Statistics and costs
- Patient advocacy
- Medical professionals

A Search site is provided to obtain information on breast cancer surgery, reconstructive surgery, and related topics. For example, regarding breast reconstruction, reports are available on:
- Mastectomy and breast reconstruction
- Federal Breast Reconstruction Law of 1998
- E-sthetics–breast reconstruction
- Patient advocate–breast reconstruction
- Olson Center for Women's Health–breast reconstruction
- Cancer BACUP–breast reconstruction
- Center for Plastic Surgery–breast reconstruction
- OncoLink- breast reconstruction
- University of Michigan Health System–breast reconstruction
- BreastDoctor.com–breast reconstruction
- BreastFlap.com–breast reconstruction
- Plastic Surgery Information Service–breast reconstruction

10.56 PubMed
http://www.ncbi.nlm.nih.gov/PubMed

PubMed (PM) is a service of the National Library of Medicine that provides access to over 11 million Medline citations dating back to the mid-1960's and additional life science journals. A Search site is provided to obtain desired information on "breast cancer" as well as related topics. PM provides abstracts of published articles on subjects searched and includes links to sites providing full text articles and other related resources for those interested. Full reference information is made available for each abstract provided for those interested in the complete report/article.

10.57 University of Wisconsin Comprehensive Cancer Center
http://www.cancer.wisc.edu

The University of Wisconsin Comprehensive Cancer Center (UWCCC) is a multidisciplinary cancer facility and a National Cancer Institute designated comprehensive cancer center. This institution is reported to be among the world's leaders in cancer research, experimental therapeutics, and medical physics (radiation therapy). Particular emphasis is placed on the evaluation of new agents, combined treatments, and cancer prevention.

Sites are provided for information on:

• Patient services

• Research and education

• Clinical trials

Breast cancer information reports available include, among others:

• Treatment and clinical trials

• Breast cancer risk assessment

• STAR study–tamoxifen versus raloxifene

A Search site is made available to search for additional information.

10.58   Wellness Community
http://www.wellness-community.org

The Wellness Community (WC), a non-profit organization, helps people with cancer and their families enhance their health and well-being by providing a professional program of emotional support, education, and hope. A full range of support services is provided in a comfortable home-like setting, completely free of charge. Drop-in and on-going support groups, networking groups for specific types of cancer, educational workshops, stress management sessions, lectures by experts in the field of oncology, and social gatherings–all with laughter, joy and hope are offered.

Information sites are featured for:
• Introduction and facilities
• Helpful info
• Patient Active concept
• Our program
• How you can help
• Cancer links

You are invited to learn about their study for women with breast cancer. This study involves five months of weekly professionally facilitated programs, either face-to-face support groups, Internet support groups, or education and stress reduction activities.

Provides an online support group for people with cancer.

10.59 Women's Health Matters Network
http://www.womenshealthmatters.ca

Women's Health Matters Network (WHMN), reported to be an evidence-based and up-to-date information source on women's health. This site is based at Women's College Ambulatory Care Centre, University of Toronto. Women's health experts from Sunnybrook and Women's College Health Sciences Centre and the Centre for Research in Women's Health developed this site and play an ongoing role in its growth. In 1996, the World Health Organization designated Women's College Hospital and the Centre for Research in Women's Health as the World Health Organization Collaborating Centre in Women's Health for the Western hemisphere.

For information on breast cancer and related topics, click on "Resources" and then on "Breast Health and Breast Cancer".

A Search site is provided to obtain additional information.

10.60 Y-Me National Breast Cancer Organization
http://www.y-me.org

Y-Me National Breast Cancer Organization (YMNBCO) was formed to decrease the impact of breast cancer, increase awareness and to insure through information, and support that no one faces the disease alone.

Information is offered in English and Spanish.

Sites are provided for information on:
- Advocacy
- Affiliates
- Breast cancer information

- News
- Special populations

Breast Cancer Profiler (BCP) provides newly diagnosed and recurrent breast cancer patients with personalized treatment information and statistics. With BCP, cancer patients can find treatment options relevant to their own diagnosis. Results allow patients and their doctors to engage in more productive and satisfying discussion and decision-making regarding treatment choices. Helps to provide information and support to patients, their families, medical professionals and the public.

A Search site is provided to obtain additional information.

ABOUT THE AUTHOR

Eugene A. De Felice, M.D., author, educator, Distinguished Clinical Professor of Medicine, Fellow of American Geriatric Society and Fellow of Academy of Psychosomatic Medicine, is listed in Marquis' 1) Who's Who in Medicine and Healthcare, 2) Who's Who in America and 3) Who's Who in the World. He is the author of 7 key medical books including "Web Health Information Resource Guide" published in 2001. The contents are outlined at http://webspawner.com/users/webhealthdoc, and available from the publisher at iuniverse.com.

0-595-22651-5

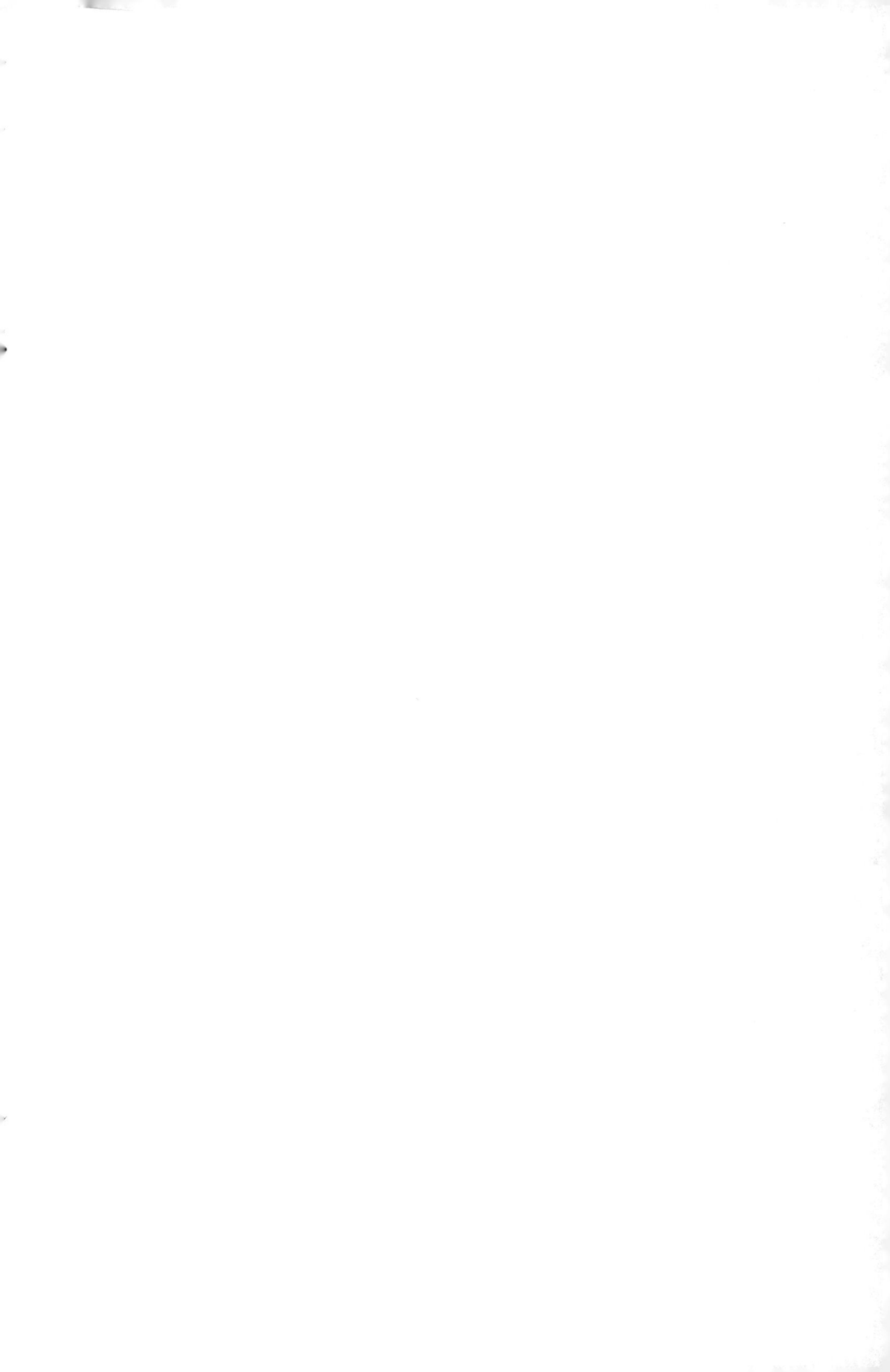